How I Survived Without Chemo Therapy

One Woman's Story from Diagnosed to Thriving

By: Sabrina Moore

Written By: Sabrina Moore

© 2018

Published in the United States by Pen Legacy
www.penlegacy.com

Distributed by IngramSpark

Edited by: U Can Mark My Word Editorial Services (www.ucanmarkmyword.com)

Cover & Interior Design by: Junnita Jackson

DISCLAIMER

Although you may find the teachings, life lessons and examples in this book to be useful, the book is sold with the understanding that neither the author nor Pen Legacy® are engaged in presenting any legal, relationship, financial, emotional, or health advice.

Any person who's experiencing financial, anxiety, depression, health, or relationship issues should consult with a licensed therapist, advisor, licensed psychologist, or any qualified professional before commencing into anything described in this book. This book's intent is to provide you with the writer's account and experience with overcoming life matters. All results will differ than yours;

however, our goal is to provide you with our "take" on how to overcome and be resilient when faced with circumstances. There are lessons in every blessing.

Library of Congress Cataloging – in- Publication Data has been applied for.

ISBN: 978-0-692-18602-2

PRINTED IN THE UNITED STATES OF AMERICA.

Table of Contents

DID YOU KNOW?

In 2018, it's estimated that among U.S. women and men there will be*:

Women

- *266,120 new cases of invasive breast cancer*

- *40,920 breast cancer deaths*

Men

- *2,550 new cases of invasive breast cancer*

- *480 breast cancer deaths*

*Susan G. Komen (2018)

Facts and Statistics
https://ww5.komen.org/BreastCancer/FactsandStatistics.html

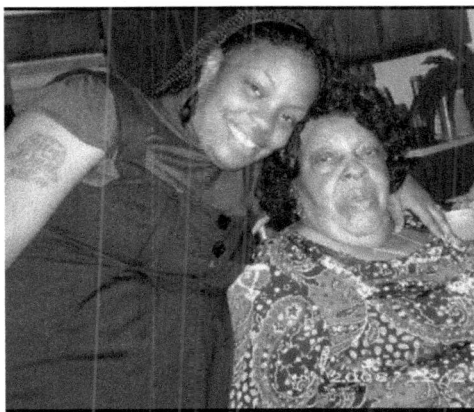

My Grandmother, Georgia M. Fletcher

Grandma, I want to say thank you. Even though I told you this many times, I just wanted to tell you again. Thank you for being the greatest role model ever, the root of our tree. You were the best grandmother to me. No matter what, you were always there when I called on you. Never once did you turn your back on me, whether I was right or wrong. If anything, you would give me a long talk about my wrongdoings, which I truly appreciated. You instilled a lot in me and taught me even more, from lessons on how to cook to teaching me about the birds and the bees. I even remember you telling me the story of the Three Little Pigs and singing your favorite grandma's baby song. I watched you care for so many people, and even on your worst days, you never showed what you were going through. You showed me how to maintain a home and how a wife is supposed to be the queen of the castle. But, the most important things you taught me were how to remain strong, to never let people see me sweat, and to never give up but instead give in. I will forever cherish these things.

After your battle with cancer and, to my dismay, losing the fight, you made me realize the true meaning of love. It's not a word that should be used if one doesn't mean it. Love is to be shown through one's actions and without the expectation of receiving anything in return. You touched the lives of many and showed plenty of people how much you loved them. When people talk about you, it's always positive words; it makes me so very happy to be attached to such a great woman like yourself.

Thank you for allowing me to care for you during your last days and for simply always loving me. I will keep your legacy alive, holding on to all my precious memories. I know without a doubt you're super proud of me for all that I have overcome and accomplished, and you're one of the reasons why. Continue to rest well, Grandma.

I love you!

Sabrina

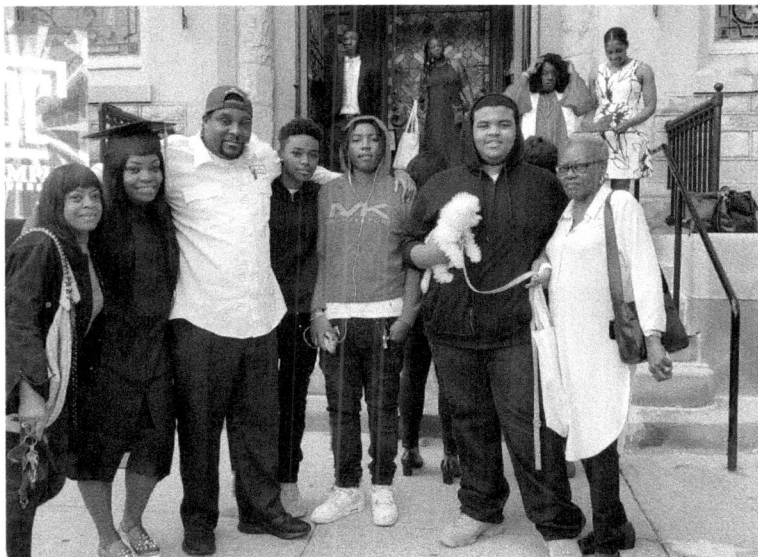

Acknowledgements

I would like to first thank my Lord and Savior Jesus Christ. To all my supporters, my family and friends, a huge thank you. Also, thanks to my sisters Erica Fletcher-Harris, Malika King, Shalika King, and Cheryl Brown; my mother, Carolyn Moore; Mom Betty King; my children, Sharell and Raquan; my aunt, Brenda Fletcher; Dante Borden; my brother and sister-in-law, Keith and Shakira Moore; my brother-in-law, Dwight Harris Sr.; Donald Council; and my nieces and nephew, DJ. Without these people, I wouldn't have made it across the finish line.

1

Prelude

Six years ago, God placed a major test upon me. Who would have thought that I, Sabrina Moore, would be faced with every woman's fear -- breast cancer. My maternal grandmother, the late Georgia Fletcher, also battled breast cancer -- two different types, which had spread to her lungs and bones. I was thirty-three years old when her health took a turn for the worse.

My grandmother and I had an unbreakable bond; she was my everything. Once she could no longer care for herself, she looked to me to take care of her. I racked my brain trying to figure out why she chose me out of all her other grandchildren. Despite whatever her reason was, before my grandmother stopped speaking, I promised her that I would take care of her until God called her home…and that's what I did.

I designed a plan for everyone who was involved in caring for my grandmother to follow while I worked. A log was kept documenting the administering of her medication and the dosage, her meals, and the name of her caregiver. The caregivers were instructed by me to document everything and include their signature. I had to make sure my grandmother was properly cared for in the comfort of her own home whenever I couldn't be there to look after her.

As the days went on, her health continued to decline. I will never forget when the hospice nurse told us that she wouldn't live through the weekend, and she didn't. On October 28, 2010, God crowned my grandmother.

Now, I would like to share my story of how I survived breast cancer without chemotherapy.

The Day the Doctor Said,
You Have Breast Cancer

Ever since I was a young girl, I was always in tune with my body. So, performing a breast exam and knowing what to feel and look for was second nature to me. Well, one Fall day in 2011, my life would change forever.

While showering, I performed my monthly exam, feeling for any lumps as I manipulated my breasts in a circular motion. I thought I was clear until I pinched my right nipple. That's where the devastation started. I had a bloody show, with old blood and new blood mixed together. Trying to stay calm, I finished washing. Afterwards, I went straight to the emergency room, where I was informed there was nothing they could do there and that I would need to see a breast specialist. That's when the anxiety started.

The next day, I called Albert Einstein Hospital to schedule an appointment to see a breast specialist. Thankfully, I didn't have to wait long and was seen within two days. Not knowing what was going on or what was about to happen, I prepared myself for whatever God had for me, whether good or bad.

During my first visit, I completed an intake form and questionnaire. After seeing the specialist, she explained the next step would be for me to have a biopsy. I was scheduled a week out. So, of course, I experienced more anxiety and anticipation while waiting. My sister, Erica, was moving from Philadelphia to Valdosta, Georgia, in two weeks or so. But, being the loving, caring, and concerned sister that she is, she stopped in the middle of her moving preparations so she could go with me to my procedure.

The day came, and we went together for me to have the in-office procedure done while I was under little sedation. After the procedure, my doctor asked for my consent to call and give me the results over the phone once she received them. Now what was I thinking when I agreed to that? Never again!

When she called with my results, I was at Quality Community Health Care, where I was currently working in the billing department. While sitting inside my cubical, my cell phone started vibrating, and when I looked down at it, I saw the number I had been anticipating receiving a call from. My heart started racing, nearly beating right through my chest wall, and I tried hard to calm myself down before answering, praying for God to give me the strength to accept whatever the doctor said. I knew whatever news awaited me on the other end of the phone could either bring relief or dismay. Not knowing which only increased my heartrate even more. Still, I knew I had to answer. My life depended on it.

"Hello, Sabrina. This is Doctor Jablon. Are you available to talk?"

"Yes," I replied.

"Is it okay to discuss your results over the phone?"

"Yes," I repeated.

"Well, we have received the results from your biopsy, and the results have determined that you have tested positive for malignant breast cancer."

6

What I had feared was now my reality!

"Okay. What stage?" I asked, void of emotion, probably because I was nearly shocked into speechlessness.

"Stage One," Dr. Jablon replied. "Most people never catch it in such an early stage, but you did because you check your breasts regularly and didn't delay in coming in to be tested."

Dr. Jablon then asked that I come into her office to discuss treatment plans, to which I agreed. At that moment, I wasn't really giving much thought to anything else she said. The only thing I could think about was death.

Before hanging up, she asked me if I had any questions. Still in shock, I told her no and that I would see her next week for my appointment.

Immediately after hanging up the phone, my brain started racing. All kinds of thoughts rushed through my head: death, my family, my children. Even after having just received the worst news of my life, I never shed a tear…well, not at that moment. I guess I had somewhat prepared myself. So, there I was. Faced with the decision to either fight to stay alive – first for myself and then for my children – or throw in the towel and die.

The first person I called after talking to the doctor was my sister, Erica.

"Sister…" I said. "My results are positive for breast cancer."

Once again, being the loving, caring, and concerned sister that she is, Erica replied, "We will get through this."

What is Breast Cancer?
My Grandmother Showed Me

My grandmother showed me how to be patience, how to care for others, and how to make sure your home is taken care of first. However, the most important thing she taught me was to stay strong and never give up! Never give up; instead give in. Those were the words she always spoke. I try to live today the way my grandmother did when she was alive, continuing to push forward daily no matter what the situation and placing my trust in God.

My grandmother, who was diagnosed with breast cancer, only had a biopsy done. She never underwent chemotherapy nor did she have surgery to remove it. She always said, "Once they cut you open, that's it. It will spread." Although diagnosed with two different types of breast cancer, my grandmother lived to be eighty years old, and I believe her decision not to have treatment helped prolong her life. The cancer eventually spread to her lungs and bones, but even then, my grandmother still pushed on, along with having other medical conditions such as COPD and emphysema. Now that's what I call a rock!

Before my grandmother's health declined to the point where she could no longer talk, feed herself, or care for herself, she expressed that she wanted me to be the one who cared for her. Again, I was puzzled as to why, out of all of her children and her grandchildren, she singled out me. Still, I made sure I fulfilled her wishes.

My grandmother was the type of person who would feed the entire block if she could. Her door was always open, and she never treated anyone better than the other. My grandmother instilled in me how to love wholeheartedly, how to always be truthful with yourself, and to never be a fool twice.

In the beginning, it was hard to see her unable to do for herself like she used to. I now had to take care of my backbone just as she had once cared for me. I often asked myself how was I supposed to do this without breaking down and falling apart. Well, prayer was my answer. I prayed and asked God daily to guide me and hold me together as I cared for my grandmother. Although it was a lot of responsibility and an extremely hard task, I couldn't break my promise to her. Knowing how many times my grandmother had rescued me from many ass whippings during my younger years, there was no way I wouldn't take care of her now. (LOL!) It was a must. No turning back, just straight forward.

After coming to an agreement and creating a plan with how everything would go concerning the caring process for my grandmother, I moved out of my house and into my grandmother's. My children went to live with my mother. With all this going on, I still managed to continue working, make sure my children went to school and their homework was completed, and cook dinner. My mother made it clear that these things had to be done in addition to caring for my grandmother, and boy, there would be some days when I would be ready to pull my hair out. I never allowed myself to break, though. Nor did I let my grandmother see how her transition was tearing me up. We never want to see our loved ones suffering or make them feel like they're a burden. So, we hide how their sickness is really affecting us. Well, at least I did.

As we prepared to celebrate my grandmother's 80th birthday and another year of blessings, she was so excited about this milestone and getting to see everyone who would be attending. This day was so special. My grandmother sang happy birthday to herself along with everyone else. It was a day filled with many good memories, and I wish I could rewind the hands of time back to that day.

When I tell you this woman who I called grandma wore her pain well, not knowing that two months after turning eighty years old she would transition over into the eternal life. She showed pain towards her last days, but she was never the type to complain. Still, I knew she was suffering.

As the cancer became more invasive, there came the need for hospice nurses. Hospice services are mainly to comfort the patient as they begin their transition from this earthly realm to a spiritual one. The nurses who cared for my grandmother were kind and compassionate. They explained what was happening step by step.

I had to turn my grandmother's dining room into an office in order to make sure she was given the best care during her last days. Since my grandmother had trouble swallowing, her medication had to be given to her in liquid form. I even had to use cotton swabs to keep her mouth moist. It was like she was reverting back to her infant days. I created a daily log, which included the amount and time of her medicine, food, and liquid intake. Her vital signs were taken daily, and we made her feel as comfortable as possible. The more my grandmother slept, the more I knew God was coming for her. I had a lot of sleepless nights just sitting up and watching her to make sure she was still breathing. I know this might sound harsh, but I used to ask God to take my grandmother because I couldn't stand the fact that she was suffering. As the days passed, her end neared. I had to prepare myself for another loss of a loved one.

Needing more support, I called on my two aunts to help out in any way that they could, and they did. My aunts would come and relieve me of my duties of caring for my grandmother so I could go to work. Before leaving, I would make sure my grandmother's medication was ready for administering and they had everything else they needed.

It was the first week in October of 2010, and we were treating each day as if it were my grandmother's last, cherishing each moment with her. My grandmother's health was steadily declining, but keeping my faith, I would tell my grandmother that I was leaving for work and would see her later. Then I would kiss her on the forehead and tell her that I loved her. Being at work wasn't easy knowing that my grandmother was on her death bed, and of course, my social life was put on hold. My grandmother was my main priority.

One night after returning home from work, I had to call the hospice nurse because of the condition and pain that my grandmother was in. The nurse instructed me to increase my grandmother's morphine and just continue to keep her comfortable, which I did.

The hospice nurse arrived on October 25, 2010, and after taking my grandmother's vitals, she told us that my grandmother wouldn't make it through the weekend. Her pulse was faint and her blood pressure was low. She advised us to gather our family and start making arrangements.

Instead of trying to process the news that I was about to lose my grandmother, all I could think about was my aunt Brenda and how I would tell her since she wasn't there when the hospice nurse informed us that my grandmother didn't have much time left. It would be the hardest thing I've ever had to do in my life. While the others didn't want to tell my aunt, I knew I couldn't let her mother just die without giving her the opportunity to spend some time with her before she left this earth. I prayed and asked God to help me stay strong and find the right words to tell my aunt what was about to happen. It brought me a little comfort that both my other aunt and my mother were present when I told her.

"Aunt Brenda," I said, "I know how much you love Grandma, and she's holding on because of you. She knows you're not ready to let her go, but the nurse told us that she will not live beyond the weekend. So, what I need you to do is go talk to her alone. She can hear you."

I hugged my aunt, then we left the room so she could have that one-on-one with her mother.

Our night was good, almost peaceful. My aunt and I watched Cooley High until we both fell asleep.

On the morning of October 28, 2010, I was moving so slow. This morning more than all the others, I didn't want to leave my grandmother and go to work. My aunt Carol came to relieve me for work, but all I kept saying was I didn't want to leave her. I was even late to work that day. Something just didn't feel right. As usual, I kissed my grandmother before leaving out, but I didn't tell her that I would see her later.

I hadn't even been at work an hour before my aunt called.

"Sabrina, I think Mommy is gone. She's not breathing."

I instantly got nervous. Thinking quickly, I told her to place a mirror under her nose to see if she was breathing, and to my relief, she was! That relief only lasted for an hour, because that's when my aunt called back to tell me that my grandmother was gone. I was all over the place. Even though I had prepared myself for the day when my grandmother would leave me, I still wasn't ready. A majority of everything I was taught about life she had taught me, and now she was gone.

I immediately returned home, and while waiting for the undertaker to come pick up her body, I still made sure she was taken care of. I wiped her face with a damp rag and closed her mouth before her body became rigid. Then I laid my head upon her chest and cried. What I was about to go through showed me how strong I was, and I didn't even realize it. You know why? Because my grandmother knew exactly what I was about to face; it just wouldn't be as intense as what she went through. But, she prepared me for my storm.

After losing my grandmother, all I had was the memories and her words of strength to live by. Even during my storm, I managed to hear her voice saying, "You got this." That's another reason why I didn't give in. Seeing what my grandmother went through and her transition had a lot to do with making me the strong woman I am today. Certain things she instilled in me prepared me for life and whatever would be placed upon my feet. Before I used to question why she chose me, but now I can say I'm grateful that I could take on the task of caring for her during her last days on earth. Not only did it prepare me mentally but also physically. It also made me understand how being strong can carry you a long way. What I have learned and will always keep in mind is that every time I have to battle something due to my breast cancer -- or any other surgeries that are needed, I always tell myself I got this. I've come too far to fail, and I have my grandmother to thank for reminding me. She was a major factor in my life and helped prepare me to weather any storm.

What is Breast Cancer?

According to Susan G. Komen, breast cancer occurs when cells in the breast divide and grow without their normal control. Tumors in the breast tend to grow slowly. By the time a lump is large enough for you to feel, it may have been growing for as long as ten years. (Some tumors are aggressive and grow much faster.) Breast cancer can begin in different parts of the breast. Breast cancer, for me, started in my right milk duct. This put me right in line with the statistic, "Between 50-75 percent of breast cancers begin in the milk ducts, about 10-15 percent begin in the lobules, and a few begin in other breast tissues." Breast cancer can spread outside the breast through blood vessels and lymph vessels. When breast cancer spreads to other parts of the body, it is said to have metastasized. There are two types of breast cancer: non-invasive breast cancer or ductal carcinoma in situ (DCIS) and invasive breast cancer.

- Non-invasive breast cancer or ductal carcinoma in situ (DCIS) occurs when abnormal cells grow inside the milk ducts, but have not spread to nearby tissue or beyond.
- Invasive breast cancer occurs when abnormal cells from inside the milk ducts or lobules break out into nearby breast tissue.

In addition, you have what is called stage IV or advanced breast cancer, or metastatic breast cancer, which is invasive breast cancer that has spread beyond the breast and axillary lymph nodes to other organs in the body (most often the bones, lungs, liver, or brain). Metastatic breast cancer is not a specific type of breast cancer, but rather the most advanced stage of breast cancer. There are plenty of ways breast cancer is treated from chemotherapy, radiation, mastectomy, or medication. Most doctors will use the medication, Tamoxifen. Tamoxifen treats women and men diagnosed with hormone-receptor-positive, early-stage breast cancer to reduce the risk of the cancer coming back (recurring) or women and men diagnosed with advanced-stage or metastatic hormone-receptor-positive disease.

Tamoxifen also causes depression, which I have been through. Another major side effect is having little to no appetite. Of course, your immune system will have a harder time fighting off colds since the body is already fighting when you have cancer.

Breast cancer is something people fear, including myself. I'm sure the first thing that anyone thinks about after being told they have cancer is death! Since I wasn't ready to die, I knew I had no other choice but to fight.

So, I did extensive research about breast cancer in order to fully understand just what kind of fight I was about to go up against. Once I understood all that I needed to know about treatment, side effects, etc., I got my mind focused. I knew this fight would take more than just physical strength. It would also require me to be strong mentally. My family and myself were willing, ready, and able to go the distance.

As I prepared myself mentally, I also had to make sure my immune system would be able to help me in this fight. Therefore, I started making some changes to my diet -- eating more vegetables and fruits, flushing my body with more water, and drinking less soda. Mentally, I shifted my thinking to more positive thoughts, and believing that God is in control, I learned to accept what I couldn't change or didn't have control over.

Living with cancer can be challenging; it will either break you or make you stronger. The outcome depends on who you are and what you will -- or will not -- allow to happen to you. The psyche plays a huge part in surviving. The more negative your thoughts, the more you start to believe your way of thinking is the correct way of living. Just know to prepare yourself for a wild hayride. Some cancers will be easier to battle than others. Depending on what stage you're in when diagnosed, you may have time to prepare like I did or you may have to just dive right in with treatment and do what the doctor thinks is best. Whatever the decision, just know there may be someone out there facing the same storm but weathering it differently.

Make sure you have the strongest support team ever, because what you don't need during this battle is a weak link. Everyone must be on the same page. Don't block out and push away the ones who are offering love and support. That's the last thing you want to do. Blocking out others only makes you go into a shell of depression, and it makes your fight tougher than it already is. Take as much time as you need to allow yourself healing time. If you need to cry, let it out. I cried many tears, and each time, it made me feel like a heavy weight had been lifted off of me. We are still human; don't you forget that.

Breast cancer tried to steal my joy and peace at an early age. I was only thirty-three years old when I was first diagnosed with it. Growing up, I always thought it only affected older people. How wrong I was! Oh, and if you have a family history of breast cancer -- or any other type of cancer, it would be a good idea to know your status. In other words, request that your doctor do genetic testing, or the BRCA1 or BRCA2 Gene. This test will determine if it's hereditary. Early detection can save your life. Don't wait until something happens to get checked out. Schedule your exams as recommended for your age, and if cancer runs in your family, get checked sooner than others.

In the last six years, I have witnessed cancer affect more and more people, both young and old. We, as humans, must stay in tune with our bodies, do self-examinations, take time to go see the doctor, and STOP making excuses! Excuses only prolong the inevitable and hurt you in the end.

I do believe that if I wasn't the kind of person who always worried about things, I wouldn't be here today to share my experience of living and being diagnosed with breast cancer in hopes that it will help and encourage others. Yes, being diagnosed is the scariest news to ever receive. Are there options? Yes. Will all of the options work? We pray that they will, but sometimes they don't. Will you get through this? Yes. Just keep in mind that our faith will be tested on a daily basis. God will test us to see how we handle it. Don't give up. Keep your faith.

Allow your support team to help you in any way they know how, and allow your voice to be heard. Your opinion counts! Don't allow others to dictate your treatment plan. Educate yourself -- if you have time -- and never regret the final decision you make. Help others that may be shelled and going through what you have already gone through.

My opinion is that breast cancer responds to how you react. If you treat it with harsh medications, it will definitely respond harshly and aggressively. Some people have no other options, so know your rights before making a life-changing decision. Talk everything over with your family as well as your doctor. Know all the side effects for whatever treatment you are considering. Most importantly, give it your all, but make sure you take some you-time so you won't mentally break down. Allow God to walk with you through this test and never ask WHY. Talking about cancer with others also helps. There are many people facing this same disease. Just don't allow the word cancer to get the best of you. Cancer is not an automatic death sentence. Fight, fight, fight, and don't give up. If anything, give in.

I Saved Myself with Self-Examination

Since breast cancer runs in my family, I began doing breast exams on myself at the age of thirteen, which is the same time that I started seeing my GYN doctor. My mother and father instilled in us the importance of taking care of our body. Being the scary type, I always thought about illnesses, diseases, and death. So, the littlest things that I would find on myself would warrant a trip to the emergency room.

Before being diagnosed with breast cancer, I had noticed some clear discharge coming from the nipple of the same breast that had the cancer in it. I went to my old job Quality Community Health Care, and the MD there told me that I shouldn't have any discharge coming from my nipples, especially if I wasn't expecting a child. She advised me to keep a watch on it. After witnessing my grandmother's experience with breast cancer, along with my maternal cousins' bouts with it, I knew I had to stay on top of the situation.

Each month after my period ended -- seven days after to be exact -- is when I would perform my own self-exams. I would start from my armpits, and in a circular motion, I would manipulate the tissue all the way to my nipple. Once I reached the nipple, I would then pinch and squeeze it to make sure there was no discharge. There wasn't any at the time.

As the months went on, I continued to do my breast exams. However, there were times when I skipped months, sometimes many months that turned into a year. Honestly, the only thing that made me start back to doing my breast exams regularly was after my grandmother was diagnosed with stage 4 breast cancer. When that happened, I knew this was serious and that I was jeopardizing myself by not being consistent. So, I started back doing my exams. Sometimes my breasts were checked twice in one month -- once by my health care provider whenever I had an appointment and the other myself. Each time I didn't discover any abnormal findings or feel any lumps, I would thank God. Yes, doing breast exams and awaiting the results of mammograms is the scariest and most nerve-racking experience, but it is necessary. Early detection plays a major part in saving your life. Stay in tune with your body and always do your monthly breast exams. One thing for certain and two things for sure, your body will definitely tell you when something is wrong. So, pay attention to the signs. Discovering it early gives you more options and a greater chance at beating it.

Another thing, I encourage ever woman to stay educated about cancer, a dreadful disease that has stolen many lives -- both young and old. Even after knowing what I knew from seeing my grandmother deal with her cancer, I still wanted to know more. Researching if cancer runs in your family, understanding the possible outcomes, and learning the steps that need to be taken if diagnosed never hurt anyone. That goes with any type of medical history. No matter what it is, get checked out. Have questions? Ask them. Still feel like you're not being provided enough information? Then do your own research and educate yourself.

Cancer doesn't discriminate. It doesn't target one particular race, age, or gender. Understand that we never know what to expect in life. Therefore, we have to take the good with the bad and vice versa. I could've died if I hadn't done my monthly breast exams and listened to my body. You cannot just do it once and, after not finding anything, think, "Okay, I'm cleared." No, no, no. That way of thinking could cost you your life. I need everyone -- not just women, but men as well -- to understand that it doesn't matter how healthy you may seem. If cancer sneaks in, it could be deadly if not treated properly and with urgency.

Make sure you educate your children both male and female about cancer and self-exams. Remember, cancer doesn't discriminate. Guys must also perform breast examinations on themselves; just because men don't have breasts, it doesn't mean they can't get breast cancer. Men, you must examine yourselves the same as women do, just not after the monthly cycle. We all know men don't have a menstrual period, but the same way a woman exams her breasts is the same way a man should examine his. Only difference is men may have to apply a little more pressure to the breast tissue in order to go deeper, and especially if they are very muscular. It's not a bad idea to practice on each other as a family, if possible, in order to learn the proper way to perform the exam. If you're uncomfortable with that suggestion, your doctor can always guide you. So, just like the women do, you will start at the armpit and manipulate the tissue in a circular motion, working it all the way down to the nipple. You can even squeeze the nipple to make sure there is no discharge. Any lumps found may be a sign of something serious that needs your attention.

But, don't panic and start to worry if there are any lumps or discharge discovered during your exam. Do make an appointment to get checked out, though.

I cannot emphasis enough what I'm about to say. Please, please, please, DO NOT stress yourself out. Stress can impact your health greatly. Oftentimes when faced with a health scare, we start to self-diagnose ourselves by reading too much about symptoms and what illness they can be directly related to. Then we start to automatically think the worst before we even get tested and receive the actual results. We read so much WebMD online that we start to think that we are an MD. Yes, it's good to do your research, but don't send yourself into a panic and think you're on your way up outta here. Get checked by a "licensed" physician, do your homework on the diagnosis in which you were informed of, and go from there.

Knowing what's going on inside your body -- and not just on the outside -- can save your life. We sometimes, myself included, only pay attention to what's going on outside the body. That's because we can't really see what's going on inside. But, knowing what's wrong inside AND on the outside helps you understand the body a lot better. Sometimes things happen to our bodies that we don't even learn about until it's too late. It's never too late to start taking steps to get your body in a healthy state.

Start by eating the right foods. Salads, fruit, baked chicken and fish are all good choices. Stay away from sodas, diet sodas included, and cut out sugar. Drink plenty of water, work out, and stay on top of any family medical history, which is another thing I can't stress enough. The family history plays an important part in you knowing who has been affected by certain diseases/illnesses, how long it's be running in your family, and if you are at risk. Just understanding helps a lot in the way you approach handling your health. You can even ask family members who are still living what steps/treatment those relatives who contracted those diseases and illnesses took; it may help you in the long run.

See, I'm the type of woman who must ask questions if I don't know something. Yes, finding out something that you really don't want to hear can be scary, but I think it's best to know what's wrong so you can decide on how to deal with it than to not know at all. Do you understand what I'm saying? Not knowing is even scarier than knowing. Not knowing leaves your mind to wander, and you can get yourself so worked up for it to turn out to be nothing. That's why I say getting a checkup is for the best, because it really is. It may or may not result in the outcome you were praying for, but at least you will know and can work towards the outcome that you want.

Knowing that breast cancer runs in my family, I would get scared at times. While doing my own exams, my heart would race, and my mind would start playing tricks on me. I told myself to calm down, and once I finished examining myself, I would thank God for not finding or feeling anything unusual. Then I would continue living my everyday life just as I did each day that the Lord allowed me to open my eyes. My days consisted of working, taking care of my kids, and simply enjoying my life. That is, until 2012.

While in the shower, I examined my breasts just like the numerous times I'd done before. However, this time when I felt around my right nipple, I noticed some bleeding. The fact that the discharge was a brownish color mixed with blood concerned me. I continued to shower, but once I got out, I did my exam once again. There was even more blood, still the same brownish-red color. At that time, I knew something wasn't right. I knew I shouldn't have any discharge -- let alone blood -- coming from my nipples.

After being diagnosed with stage 1 breast cancer, I was faced with having to make some major decisions and do a lot of research. It was a very stressful, and I prayed that I would make the right decision. Not only that, but I prayed I would be able to accept whatever decision I chose. Then there was having to make sure my children understood exactly what we were about to face. Even though I didn't know whether my decision would turn out to be a good or bad thing for me, I knew I had to stick with whatever I said. I couldn't doubt or second-guess anything. I prayed for the Lord to place me on the right track and then got ready for the ride.

After talking everything over with my family, my mother said to me, "I think you have made the right decision." At that moment, I knew I had the best support team ever and that we would defeat this together.

I started the process at my job to take FMLA, which is a family medical leave. This way, my position would be protected while I was out on leave. With no emergency funds saved, I took advantage of all the help from family, friends, support groups, and organizations I could possibly take. I knew the fight wouldn't be easy, but fighting was the best option I had. After all, I couldn't give up. I couldn't let cancer get the best of me.

I know I keep saying this, but I need everyone who is reading this book to understand that having a routine breast cancer screening is the best thing you can do for yourself. Even if you don't have any symptoms or there are no serious health issues that run in your family, still consider getting tested. Do it for yourself if not for anybody else. Life is too precious, and God gave us this life to fight no matter how hard it gets.

For everyone who is struggling with this disease, know that there is a light at the end of the tunnel. You have to want to fight see it. Keep fighting to reach it until you can't fight no more, and even then, keep going.

I knew my fight wasn't over, and I wasn't going to stop for nothing. A child of God, I was too strong to just lay down and let this cancer get the best of me.

Since early detection is the best detections, below is a step by step guide on how a Breast Self-Exam be performed, according to National Breast Center. (https://www.nationalbreastcancer.org/breast-self-exam)

1) In the Shower

Using the pads of your fingers, move around your entire breast in a circular pattern moving from the outside to the center, checking the entire breast and armpit area. Check both breasts each month feeling for any lump, thickening, or hardened knot. Notice any changes and get lumps evaluated by your healthcare provider.

2) In Front of a Mirror

Visually inspect your breasts with your arms at your sides. Next, raise your arms high overhead. Look for any changes in the contour, any swelling, or dimpling of the skin, or changes in the nipples. Next, rest your palms on your hips and press firmly to flex your chest muscles. Left and right breasts will not exactly match—few women's breasts do, so look for any dimpling, puckering, or changes, particularly on one side.

3) Lying Down

When lying down, the breast tissue spreads out evenly along the chest wall. Place a pillow under your right shoulder and your right arm behind your head. Using your left hand, move the pads of your fingers around your right breast gently in small circular motions covering the entire breast area and armpit. Use light, medium, and firm pressure. Squeeze the nipple; check for discharge and lumps. Repeat these steps for your left breast.

Also note, a mammography can detect tumors before they can be felt, so screening is key for early detection. But when combined with regular medical care and appropriate guideline-recommended mammography, breast self-exams can help women know what is normal for them so they can report any changes to their healthcare provider.

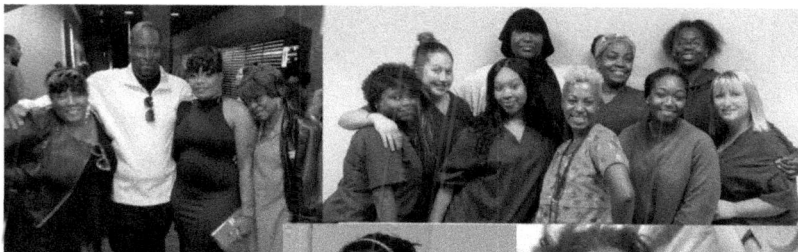

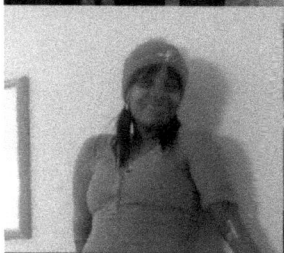

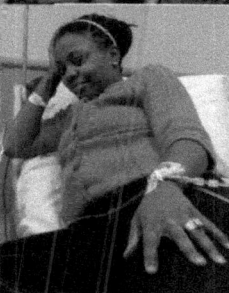

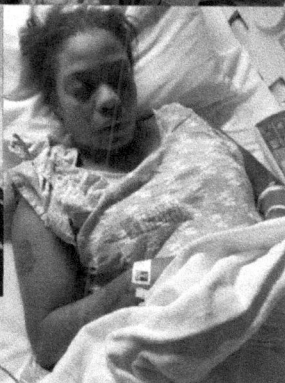

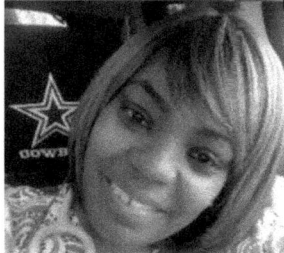

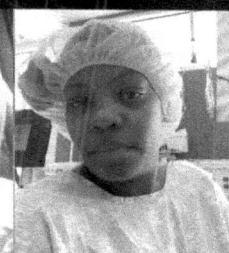

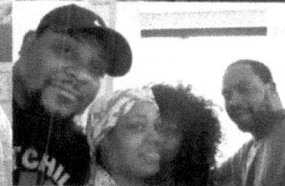

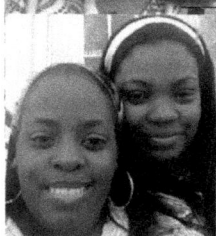

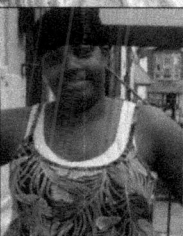

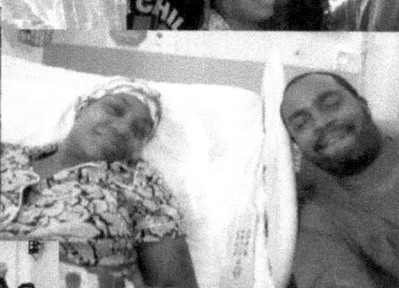

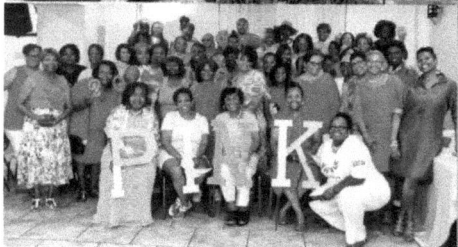

DEAN'S LIST AWARD

THIS CERTIFICATE IS AWARDED TO

Sabrina Turner

In recognition of Outstanding Academic Achievement during
the July 9, 2018—August 19, 2018 Academic Module.

Am I Going to Die? Options, Please

Am I going to die? I asked myself that question over and over, time and time again. Living with breast cancer is one thing to worry about, but then there are the thoughts of death, of which I had many. Am I going to beat this or will I die? I knew I couldn't just ignore this question; I knew one day I would have to talk about my fears. The thought of dying has been in my mind since the minute I found out I had breast cancer. It's a hard pill to swallow. Truly, it is. I cried more times than I can remember.

Looking over my life was something I found myself doing often. I asked myself if I had done everything I wanted to do, or did I not do enough. I sat alone with my thoughts at times, thinking about the outcome. One thing I did know is that I was going to put up the best fight I could, fight to live.

But, what if my best isn't good enough? What if God says, "Sabrina, I'm calling you home to ease your pain. With me, you will be free."

Now, I'm not going to lie. The thought of being free from the stress and pain that I knew my body would endure made me feel like I would welcome returning to my God if

He called me home. Then I thought about my kids, my family, my friends, and the life I would be leaving behind. That wouldn't be fair to them if I just give up, I thought to myself. But what if I didn't have a choice? After all, undergoing any surgery puts you at risk of dying. Looking back, I could've died on that operating table while having the mastectomy or in the hospital room after the surgery when I started having complications. But, the truth is, I wasn't ready. I'm pretty sure no one is ever ready to die. Not unless you're one of those people who want to choose the way you will die. Not me, though. I wasn't ready at all, but who am I to question God and what he does? Let's face it. I didn't have control over when I entered this world, and I don't get to decide when I will leave here. God is in total control of all that. Whenever He is ready to take me, He will. I can't just tell Him, "No, I'm staying." I don't possess that type of power; only He does. So, it was His choice if he called for me.

If I can be transparent for a moment, I'm scared of the thought of dying. I feel like I still have so much more of me to give. I know my road is going to be a long one, and honestly, I'm ready to walk it. I'm ready to do whatever I need to do to kick cancer's ass.

See, the one thing about having cancer is that it affects everyone differently. There are some who catch it in time, and unfortunately, there are others who are diagnosed in later stages. Cancer steals many lives each year. Young, old. Black, white. Men, women. It doesn't matter. However, the ones who catch it in time with early detection have greater survival odds and a better chance of fighting it.

Depending on the stage of cancer when one is diagnosed, it will determine if the person will need to learn the right way to fight it so they can live, or if they will fight to live only long enough to put things in order. Knowing that not receiving the proper treatment would put me in danger of dying made me grow closer to the man upstairs.

Now, there are some people who instead of running towards God in this time, they turn away from Him. Some grow angry with God. Some might question if God is real, debating that if He is real, why does he allow such sickness and suffering. Well, I can't speak for everyone else. But, as for me, I turned to Him to help me find the peace I needed to deal with this. Because without him, I would've given up. I would've let this disease take me away from everything and everyone.

I'm often asked how do I stay so strong knowing what I'm facing? And my answer is always the same: My faith in God. I'm scared every day knowing that the cancer can return once it's removed, and knowing this makes me even more afraid of the outcome of things. However, I must focus all my energy on living and not entertain the thought of dying. I must do all that I can to stay alive. It's not easy, but I have to do my best. I will continue to fight every day if it means not letting cancer win. I'm too strong to just give in. I love life too much to just throw in the towel.

I encourage anyone who is dealing with breast cancer -- or any other cancer or disease --to ask themselves the same question I asked myself: Am I going to die? Then think long and hard about your answer, and be honest with yourself. Because if u choose to fight, you have to be willing to deal with the changes your body will go through. You must be willing to live a different lifestyle than what you were accustomed to living. You must fight harder every day and prove to not only yourself but to others that if you can beat cancer, anyone else can, as well.

With any new diagnosis of a life-threatening disease, the thought of you dying will surely cross your mind and will more than likely remain there until you get through whatever you're facing. For me, the closest I came to death was having an out-of-body experience after having my surgery. Till this day, I still think about death, and it literally scares me to tears. Yes, I know we all have to die one day, but who wants to die from any painful disease, especially cancer. From the moment that I was diagnosed with it, all I could think about was death and who would care for my children after I was gone. With both of my children being too young to fully understand death, I knew I had to put up the biggest fight of my life. Still, there were times when I thought there was no chance for me to survive and feared the worst. Every time I had to go for any special tests, death crossed my mind. When faced with having to make a decision concerning my treatment, I knew the right choice had to be made or else my chances of surviving would be slim to none.

Death is a touchy conversation. Most people would rather not talk or even think about death, so they aren't prepared for it. As for myself, I had to be prepared and also prepare my family by getting things in order just in case I was called home. I didn't want my loved ones to have to struggle with trying to gather money for my funeral expenses. So, I got all my affairs in order to elevate the stress off my family. In my opinion, most people should indeed do the same and preferably before tragic strikes. As the saying goes, better to be safe than sorry. So, talk with your loved ones about your plan and don't let this be something that you put off doing. Make it a priority. We don't know the day nor the hour when our Father will call us home. So, just be prepared.

What I'm saying might sound harsh, but the fact is there are two things guaranteed in life: we are born and we will die. Death is something we will all have to face; there's no hiding from it. If you don't have life insurance, seek information about it. Get it before any sickness occurs. I'm only telling you this from experience. I was turned down by insurance companies because of my medical history. However, there will always be one that will accept you regardless. Also, have a living will done. These things are so important. Do them while you are still able and in your right state of mind. After witnessing what I did after losing my grandmother, I knew for a fact that I did not want my children to be fighting over messy business, and neither should you. Take care of your business before your calling.

I am truly -- and I do mean this with every breath in me -- truly grateful that I was given a second chance at life. Just remember that with life comes death, and with death, hearts will be broken. Thinking about death doesn't make you creepy or weird. It just shows a sign of maturity. It also lets God know that your faith is unwavering and that you accept death as a part of life. Now, live life, don't overthink the process, continue to fight, and be beautiful.

Chemo or No Chemo?
That Was the Question

After being told that I had breast cancer, I was faced with having to make the biggest decision ever – to have chemotherapy or decline it. I decided to step out on my faith and decline chemotherapy. I knew undergoing chemotherapy would hurt me more than help me. Want my opinion on chemotherapy? Well, here it is.

Chemotherapy is a harsh regimen with many different medicines combined in it from Adriamycin, Taxotere, Cytoxan, and Taxol. These are just a few medicines that some may use depending on the cancer's stage and location. Anthracyclines is a chemical that damages the genetic cancer cell. Taxanes interfere with the way cancer cells divide in the location.

Technically, chemotherapy works by slowing or stopping the growth of the cancerous cells. The treatment can be very intense. Cycles can last from two hours to one or more days. Normally, the patient has to undergo four to six cycles over a six-month period.

What concerned me was how it actually damages the body and all of the side effects, which include fatigue, hair loss, easy bruising and bleeding, infection (especially with a stent in place), anemia (which I already have), constipation, loss of appetite, nausea, and vomiting. Within six hours of having a treatment, the patient's skin may darken but then return to its normal color in about ten to twelve weeks. It may cause lesions in the mouth; this is caused by damaged cells in the lining of the mouth. The person may also experience neuropathy, which is nerve damage that often occurs in the hands and feet -- causing numbness, weakness, and sometimes a decreased sex drive.

With all of these side effects, I never gave it a second thought. In addition to worrying about all of the side effects, I thought about Kenny, my significant other at the time, and how it would affect him. When your significant other is by your side, they have to be just as strong as you. I didn't want to go through it for myself, and I certainly didn't want to put him through it. I was already mentally broken down from the devastating news; I felt like the biggest bricks were being thrown at me at once. So, when chemotherapy was mentioned as an option during a conversation with my doctor, I replied with an emphatic NO!

"Remove my breast," I told her.

"But you're so young," she said. "And you may want to have more children."

"Well, if God decides to bless me with more children, they can be bottle fed," I replied back.

I'm sure my doctor would have loved for me to have gone along with her and started chemo. After all, it would've helped keep her pockets padded. But, it wasn't something that I thought would cause more harm to me than good, so I declined.

Even after informing my doctor of my decision, she asked me if I was sure. I thought I had made myself very clear, but after I gave her the look of death, she knew then that chemotherapy was not an option and to cross it off her list so she wouldn't make the mistake of ever bringing it back up to me again.

Having to deal with the stress of having cancer was enough; I didn't need the added stress of having to deal with all the side effects of chemo. Nope, chemotherapy was not for Sabrina. I was determined to survive without having chemo, and six years later, I'm still kicking it.

I've seen many people's life span cut short after having chemotherapy. In my opinion, this regiment only slows down the process. Basically, it may kill some cells, but surely not all of them. If it did, then why does it come back? And sometimes more aggressively than before in a different area. So now, the person has to go through another process of having more rounds of chemo. These are my questions and concerns about chemotherapy.

When I think about chemo, I think about being sick and losing weight. Those two things alone turned me off and pushed me to seek other treatment options. Now, I know some people will have no other choice but to have chemotherapy treatment. My suggestion to those people is to build your immune system before starting treatment. Take a daily multivitamin, eat more vegetables (especially kale greens), stay away from other people who may be sick, wash your hands and cover your mouth when coughing or sneezing.

When cancer enters our body, it attacks our immune system. Our body will try to fight it off because that's what it is designed to do. Since cancer patients' immune systems are weak, it's harder for our body to fight. Chemo kills not only the bad cells but some of the good cells, as well. This is just something to keep in mind if you have no other option but chemotherapy.

Also, plan out your days ahead of time so you won't get sidetracked or start to feel overwhelmed with the process, and take everything in slowly. Ask questions. You need to educate yourself about the drug and what to expect. I know people tend to not follow the doctor's orders, but in this case, please do. Drink plenty of water and keep a diary of any changes you may experience. Last but certainly not least, make sure you include a family member so they can be involved every step of the treatment.

Chemo wasn't for me, but it doesn't mean it will be the best decision for you. My advice to anyone who is undecided about whether or not to undergo chemotherapy is to weight all of your opinions and educate yourself. If your cancer was caught in the early stage like mine, you can afford the time to look into other options so you can decide on the one that will be best for you. You must understand that this your life, and only you will have to deal with the side effects, possible damage it may cause, mental disturbance, and self-esteem issues that may result from having chemotherapy. Be prepared for everything that may come with this treatment. Ask yourself if chemo is right for you or if you can beat this without it. What are your chances of survival with receiving chemo versus how long will you live after chemo? Other people's opinions about your decision should make no difference to you. This is your life! Do whatever it takes to keep living, and if you feel like stepping out on faith is one of those things, then go for it. Look at me! I did! So, never underestimate the power of yourself and stand on the word of God.

Mastectomy? Take Two!

Hello, Mastectomy! Yes, that's the treatment I chose. I had other options, but after doing my research, I felt it was the best decision for me. The only thing is, most times the person only has one breast removed. Well, I had a double bilateral prophylactic mastectomy with free flap reconstruction, which included a tummy tuck along with liposuction and removal of my right axillary sentinel lymph node. My breast was removed off of the pectoralis muscle from superior-to-inferior and from medial-to-lateral. This included the pectoralis fascia. My word of advice to anyone who plans to undergo a surgery of any kind is to educate yourself about the procedure beforehand. Trust me, it will bring you some level of comfort, if not totally.

Before my surgery was performed, I had to see a psychiatrist, and yes, I would advise that everyone see one because this type of surgery will lower your self-esteem and raise your level of depression. My psychiatrist performed several tests to make sure I was mentally prepared for what I would go through before, during, and after the procedure. After passing the required tests, I was ready to schedule the surgery.

Having done my homework and discussed the procedure with my doctor extensively, I knew what to expect. Also before going under the knife, I met with my plastic surgeon and breast surgeon multiple times to make sure we were all on the same page. I made sure I created a rapport with my surgeons. After all, I was placing my life in both of their hands. So, why wouldn't I?

Once I received my surgery date, I knew there was no turning back. I had to keep moving forward. I continued to educate myself about what I would go through before and after surgery, and how I would have to change my lifestyle after a double mastectomy. I talked everything over with my family, and let me tell you, I couldn't have been more blessed with awesome supporters. My family never once tried to get me to change my mind; they always stood behind my decisions.

May 29, 2012. The day of my surgery finally arrived, and I was more than ready. My sister Erica and a friend of mine at the time named Kenny were there with me. While being prepped for surgery, once again thoughts of death rushed my mind, but I combated my fears with faith and prayer. After the surgical site markings were placed on me, I laid there patiently waiting to go into the operating room. I used the time to pray and thank the Lord for even bringing me this far.

Both my breast and plastic surgeons came in to see me before it was time to say my farewells to my family. They again explained to me in detail what I was going to have done.

"Okay, Sabrina," my breast surgeon said, "we're going to make an upper abdominal incision as well as lower abdominal incision and dissect the flaps. Then we'll dissect out your lateral row muscle, sparing free TRAM flaps on both sides of my hemiabdomen. The flaps will be split on the midline and inserted for completion."

Ready or not, the time had come, and I was wheeled to the operating room. Once in the OR, I was asked several questions. This was done to make sure I was in my right state of mind. Then, in a blink of an eye, I was put under general anesthesia.

After being in surgery for nearly ten hours, my first thought after waking up in the recovery room was, I made it. Thank you, God, for your mercy. From the recovery room, I was moved to a private room. Now, this is where it gets a little touch and go.

Although all I wanted to do was take a nap after undergoing such an intense surgery, it was not to be. The beeping of the machines that measured my vitals alerted the nurses that something was wrong. My heart rate and blood pressure were sky high and they couldn't get either of them under control. Well, of course, here comes the doctor. So, I'm thinking to myself, This must be serious!

The doctor explained, "Okay, Sabrina, we're trying to get your vitals stable. Your left breast pulse is very faint, and we need it to be stronger so we don't have to rush you back into the OR and completely remove that breast."

Lord, help me!

My doctors and nurses, who were excellent, continued to work to get my vitals back within a normal range. During this time, I had an out-of-body experience.

Yep, you read right. Now, I have always heard of people having an out-of-body experience, but I had never experienced it for myself until then.

While the doctors and nurses were doing all they could to help me, and my sister and Kenny were standing at the foot of my bed, I looked up from where I was lying ...and saw myself behind them. How could that be? I was looking down at myself and watching the doctors take care of me.

Just as I said to my sister, "Don't let them take me, Erica", things started to return to normal. Of course, my sister couldn't remember me saying a word to her. That's because I was the one having the out-of-body experience, not her.

What a wake-up call! Immediately, I knew I had to change some things about myself, because I received a message from God that day. Basically, what He told me -- without actually having to say it -- was that he could've taken me home with him, but instead, he was giving me a second chance at life. To this day, I never take anything for granted. Just one wake-up call will have you thinking and living differently. Well, at least for me it did.

Thankfully, I didn't have to be rushed back into the OR. Finally, I was able to rest and try to wrap my mind around everything I had just gone through.

Now, let's talk about the pain. I was in so much pain, wrapped from the top of my breasts all the way to the bottom of my abdomen. Oh, and let me not forget to mention those good ole Jackson Pratt drains, known as JP drains. Ugh! Those things are the worst. The drains are placed so blood won't form any blood clots, and they allow fluid to be released. I had four drains, one on each side of my breasts and two in my groin area. For two to three weeks, these drains had to be stripped and the fluid measurements logged daily to make sure the appropriate amount of fluid was being released. Once the fluid level dropped below 25 ml per day, the drains would be removed.

Day 2 took me by surprise. I was actually able to walk around, when only the day before I could barely move in the bed. I guess when you're determined, nothing can stop you. You should have seen the facial expressions of the nurses as I walked around their station. They couldn't believe I was so mobile after having such a major surgery. One nurse's exact words were, "We've never had a patient up and walking the next day after having the type of surgery you had. It normally takes about three days for a patient." I told y'all I was determined to live!

I stayed in the hospital for a week. Once discharged, I stayed at my mother's house, where I knew I would be well taken care of. My daughter, who was only thirteen years old at the time, spent her entire summer helping me. She would wash me daily, help me to the bathroom, and even wipe my backside. And my sister, Erica, was the best nurse ever. She never once left my side. Whatever I needed, she was there to provide. My entire family was such a major help.

Visiting nurses came out to make sure my dressings were being changed properly and to keep an eye on my blood pressure. My nurse had to teach my sister how to strip my JP drains and record my fluid levels. When I tell you Erica was phenomenal during all of this. She even made a lymphedema sleeve for me after my arm swelled up like a blowfish as a result of the nurse mistakenly taking my blood pressure on the wrong arm. Lymphedema is when the fluid is not moving well. Since I had to have my lymph nodes removed from my right arm, that arm should no longer be used for blood pressure readings, blood draws, etc. So, for anyone who has had their lymph nodes removed from their arm, please remember that whichever arm they were taken from is no longer available for use. It would be best to wear a bracelet indicating this in case of an emergency and so it won't be done in error. Lymphedema may cause you to experience the following symptoms: pain that radiates from your shoulders down your arm, a feeling of tenseness, and tight discomfort. This can last anywhere between two to twelve weeks. Treatment includes complete decongestive therapy (CDT) for one hour and foam bandages worn for twenty-three hours per day. To avoid this, prior to having your blood pressure taken or blood drawn, make sure you inform doctors, nurses, and other medical assistance staff that you've had your lymph nodes removed.

Facing recovery, I didn't think the road would be so hard. After being cut from hip to hip and having a tummy tuck, I couldn't walk without the assistance of a walker. And whenever I tried to stand up straight, it felt like my skin was going to tear apart. This discomfort lasted for about two weeks; however, with each day that passed, I gradually started being able to stand in a more upright position. For three weeks, I encountered sleepless nights, even with the Dilaudid I was taking for pain. On top of the anxiety I was experiencing from wondering how I looked under the bandages, I also went through a deep depression stage and had a mental breakdown. Who was there to catch me during my low point? You guessed it. My sister, Erica!

From my previous conversations with my psychiatrist prior to having the surgery, I knew there was a great chance I would have to battle depression, but can one ever be truly prepared to go through it? We always think we can handle certain situations until we are actually facing them. This depression took me through stages of anxiety where one minute I wanted to see how I looked and then the next minute I was telling myself I wasn't ready. I even questioned God, asking him why me. But, in the same breath, I thanked him for saving my life, remembering how I had lost my grandmother, other family members, and some friends to cancer.

By not being able to work and having nothing really to do until I recovered, it left me with plenty of time to think. While my brain was trying to play catch up with my body's reality, it slowed my recovery. It had not sunk into my brain, but my body had already accepted the change. Once my brain and my body were on the same page, I was able to finish my recovery.

Two weeks post-op, and it was time for my first follow-up visit with my surgeon. It was also the day I thought I would have my JP drains removed. Well, you can imagine my disappointment when my doctor told me that my fluid level was still above the normal levels, and therefore, my JP drains needed to stay in an extra week. I was looking forward to having them removed, but then I figured I had made it that far, so another week wouldn't hurt me.

Well, that week went by slower than molasses, and my anxiety was high during that entire time. I wanted those drains OUT! When the day finally came, I felt a tremendous amount of relief and could rest better. Without the drains, I was able to walk without the use of a walker. Then, came the moment of truth. It was time to see how my breasts looked after reconstruction.

I must say both surgeons did an outstanding job! I thought I would look horrible, but overall, I was quite pleased with the outcome, even with my missing areola and nipples -- which I had to go back to have done. My areola was tattooed on by my plastic surgeon, and my nipples were formed by pulling up the skin of my breasts and stitching it. Pretty cool, huh? I have no sensation in my breasts, though. They are soft like breasts, but there is no feeling and I get no pleasure from someone touching them. Sucks, right? But, I'm still alive, and that's what matters the most.

My tummy tuck had me looking like a teenager again, flat stomach and all. My love handles, however, still hung from my sides like dog ears. I had to have a liposuction procedure done to remove the fat from those areas. Of course, with each procedure you undergo, you put your both through more stress. So, I had to be patient and space it out.

My liposuction procedure was done in an outpatient setting while I was under general anesthesia. Liposuction is the contouring of the body. Small incisions were made on my stomach area and a cannula inserted into the fatty areas between the skin and muscle. Excess fat is removed through the cannula using a suction pump or large syringe.

After the procedure, I went home but was extremely sore, tender, and bruised from all the stabbing and poking. In spite of all the procedures I had to undergo, the outcome remains the same today: I'm alive, able to share my experience, and encouraging others by telling my story.

The fight isn't going to be easy. Yes, you will cry, and yes, you will want to throw in the towel. But, keep pushing! Don't allow stress to overpower you and block your path to victory. Talk to others that may have experienced what you are going through. Those who may have never gone through what you are facing may not fully understand, but talk to them about it anyway. Don't think you're different from others or that people may judge you because of your illness. You're still human, so let your voice be heard. The same way I'm encouraging others by getting my message out, please do the same.

Every recovery is different. Having a mastectomy made me aware of some other health issues that I have recently found out about over these past years. I have been diagnosed with alpha thalassemia, which is a blood disorder that reduces the production of hemoglobin. I'm missing two of the mutations in the alpha globin genes. This led to me having to see a hematologist-oncologist to have weekly infusions done. It wouldn't be my last procedure, but guess what? I was ready for more. Why? Because I'm a fighter.

Thrive, Survive, New Perception on Life

How my thrive turned into me surviving. Man, I've come a long way with this journey. From the start even until now, I have learned the importance about life and how precious it is. Being in between a rock and a hard place will definitely change your entire aspect on life. I have grown and become humbler. Within these past years, I went from thinking I was untouchable and nothing could ever happen to me (until cancer struck), to not taking for granted the gift of breath given by God. If nothing else could change my life, this did. It made me cherish life and appreciate others. It even made me cherish how I spent my time, and I started to forgive and stop judging others.

Yes, I lost some people, even friendships, during all this. Unfortunately, I learned the hard way, but my thrive made me into the survivor I am today. Who knows where or what I would be doing today if I never had to fight for my life. Staying alive was my main focus. Therefore, certain things in my life had to be changed. So, that's exactly what I did. I made some changes. I had to eliminate the bad -- negative thoughts and actions, and even negative people -- and replaced it with good. Even when people tried to slander my name or assassinate my character, I let them be. Before, I would have been at their house, job, etc. But, this journey has indeed brought out the best of me, even with the situation being bad. All bad things aren't bad, and all good things aren't good. Sometimes you must know the difference and weigh your options before jumping out of the plane.

My new perception on life has brought me closer to God than ever before. There was a time when I was all over the place, in between religions, not knowing which way to go. I couldn't really find myself or even know where to start. I realize now that God had to place me in a storm in order to get my full attention, and if I had to do it all over again, I would do just that because I know my faith in Him will always have me coming out a winner in the end. In my new life, I have made many changes and accomplished some goals that I only talked about before but never put forth any effort to achieve. Look at me now! I'm pursuing my career and have gone back to school to get my BSN (Bachelor of Science in Nursing) so I can accomplish my goal of being the head nurse in hospice. My desire is to help others and their family when they are facing death. Yes, loved ones need to be comforted and put at ease, too. That's where I'll come into play. I want to be the one who will walk with the family during this hardship and their loved one's transition of life.

Looking back at everything I've been through, I know this next journey will be challenging, but it's nothing I won't be able to overcome. I know my calling is to help others. I have to live this new life like it's my last breath. The first life that I was given was already returned and exchanged for this new one. I must follow my ordered steps and never turn back. I'm walking with a purpose in life now, and I will never take life for granted nor will I doubt death. I promised myself that I will not stress over things that I have no control over. I will allow my past to keep me moving forward. After all, it's my past that made me who I am today: strong, determined, and focus. I'm a survivor. It's the best feeling ever, and now that I've won this fight, I can help others with theirs, as well.

As I walk in this new life, my journey will continue to take me where I want to be, without the ignorance or knowledge of any roadblocks along my path. I will be able to handle obstacles better now than before. For me, thriving is to continue to shine through the clouds, be all that I can be, and continue to keep God first. Being a survivor, I will continue to live according to my purpose in life, remain focused during my journey, accomplish my remaining goals, help those who need my help, and continue to fight with those who have chosen to fight this alone.

I have turned over a new leaf, and as I move closer to turning forty years old, I'm looking forward to all that awaits me in this new chapter. I'm so ready to speak to all groups of people on how important it is to educated themselves about cancer, how it effects your life, and the correct way to perform self-exams. Sometimes cancer doesn't show any symptoms until the later stages, but if you do have signs, it's very important to take action immediately. I want people to stop living in silence and start speaking more about their experience. You never know how your story might help the next person. My survival has taught me how to bloom like the rose that I am and to not allow negative words to dictate my destination. Stay strong! Giving up is weakness.

I will never allow what I've been through to be an excuse to keep me from doing what is best for me. I will continue to walk with my head held high in this new body that has been transformed from having a double mastectomy, breast reconstruction, liposuction, a breast lift, fat grafting, and a tummy tuck. I did not undergo all these procedures with the goal of having a new body. All the pain and recovery that I endured was the sacrifice I made to save my life. Behind every scar, I have a story to tell.

I love sharing my story with others, then seeing the reaction on their face when I tell them what I've been through. You would think I was the first person ever to be diagnosed with breast cancer. The first thing they say is, "Oh my God! I'm so sorry." And my reply is always, "Why? I'm not. It has made me into a humbler person." I now know how to accept things in life and thank God for all my blessings – both good and bad. When I talk about being a survivor, it makes me smile. My heart skips a beat knowing that at one point in time, I didn't have a clue whether or not I would live or die. I had to face the possibility that I might have to leave my young children and worried who would care for them the same way that I do as their mother. But, to God be the glory! I'm still here today. So, every chance I get to share my story, I will do just that.

Every year, I look forward to Breast Cancer Awareness Month so that I can acknowledge others who have not been as blessed as myself. Even though my awareness is every day, it is especially heightened during the month of October. I will continue to keep my Pink sisters alive; I will remind others and support my Pink sisters.

I have met so many wonderful people -- both women and men – who are battling cancer, and they are such awesome people. My recent connection was this past summer when I was honored to be a guest speaker at a Pink affair. The turnout was huge, and I was able to share my story. Some of the people may have gone through what I went through, while I'm sure there were other who were just starting their fight. The love that these women showed me, you would have thought we've known each other for years. So now, I am a Pink sister, as well, and I will continue to attend as many events as I can.

The best part about being a thriving survivor is the new perception you have on life. I'm able to accept the new me and love myself even more in order to love others. My self-esteem has taken me to another level of confidence. I feel like I'm walking on air. I can't even walk past a mirror without taking a picture. Aside from my new perception on life, my current love life is one of the best I've experienced prior to my previous relationship in which I was married. Of course, I divorced him, but there is no bad blood between us. I'm looking forward to enjoying every new thing that I have encountered and celebrating every hurdle that I have overcome. I am truly grateful.

This walk has been interesting. I've had my bad days and some good days, as well. I've gotten better at dealing with my depression, and moving forward, I will continue with the proper care -- with the end goal being that I will no longer be labeled as having depression. I expected that this part of my journey would take longer, and while I'm no doctor, my assumption would be that it's taking longer because I went through so many different procedures. As a result, my mental hasn't caught up with all of my physical changes. How funny is that!

My depression isn't fully under control, but I wear it well and try not to let it interfere with work or my relationship with my family. But, you also have to remember that there are levels to depression. My depression isn't at a major level, not like it was in the beginning. I only talk to my therapist when I feel like I can't control the depression. That's normally only after I've been feeling down for two or more days or when I start to feel like it may be getting the best of me. I was taught how to nip it before it gets too bad, and a majority of the time, I know how to convert my depression at onset. Yoga and deep breathing techniques have helped me tremendously. Again, these suggestions may or may not work for you, but they are options. Find what helps you when dealing with depression. I will say this, though. Don't allow your depression to continue for too long without seeking help. Get help before it totally damages you!

You Are Not Alone! Can I Help You?

As I said before in previous chapters, having support is essential during your fight. You need the support to weather this storm. As humans, we all have a breaking point at some time. Some things aren't doable alone, and this is one of them. Talking about what you are going through with others can help with learning how to cope with what is going on. I have been in your shoes and want to help anyone who may not have family -- or have a family they can't turn to -- and need an ear to just vent. Having cancer is already tough to deal with, but having to fight it alone makes it even more complicated. Allow me to walk with you during this journey.

Experience is a good teacher, and I'm willing to use the knowledge and wisdom that I gained from my past experiences to help others. Don't allow fear -- or pride -- to keep you from being helped. There are people out there who might be going through what you are or something even more intense. Each battle will be different; no two people go through the exact same pain or experience. Allow someone to hug you, talk to you, comfort you. Although I can't take the pain away, I can help you cope with it. I can educate you as much as I can and even be your support during a doctor's visit. Moral support is needed not just for your mental state but for your physical state of being, as well. So, please know you are not alone!

I have been down this road, and I know it isn't easy. The uncertainty of not knowing where this journey may take you or what path you may end up on is enough to drive you to the edge. But, hold on. Don't give up.

As for myself, my kids are my motivation to keep fighting every day. I've changed so much since learning that I had cancer. I changed my eating habits, started working out more, and taught myself everything I needed to know about continuing life after my battle with cancer. Whatever you do, don't get sad or worry. I know it's going to be hard, but try not to stress yourself out. Trust that everything will be just fine.

While battling cancer, I believe there are some things you should do. You should journal, write a daily entry. Good or bad, happy or sad. It doesn't matter. Write down everything you're feeling on that day. If you start to experience any emotional changes that you just can't seem to get a grip on, talk with your doctor. Again, stress can hinder your healing. Stay active. Get up every day and do something. Do not let this disease bring you down or keep you from doing the things you like to do. Live your life the best way you know how. If I can do it, so can you. Just don't give up. Fight every day and go harder than you've ever done before. Taking care of yourself is a must. Eat right, get enough sleep, and relax your mind.

Another important thing is to not isolate yourself. Open up and talk about what's going on with you. It doesn't matter if it's your mother, father, sister, brother, boyfriend, girlfriend, friend or foe. Share how you're feeling with someone who you know will listen and ask questions if they don't understand. Have that one supportive person who's always going to be there for you, no matter the day or time.

This disease will make you look at a lot of things and people differently. You will go through a wide range of emotions. More times than not, you will get easily upset. But, try to keep a positive attitude. Yes, it's going to be hard. Especially when you come across those people who think they know what's best for you, how you should feel, or what you should be doing. There will be times when you just want to tell them to shut the hell up. That you're the one living with this disease, not them. Don't do that, please. Instead, listen to what they have to say. I mean, even a broken clock tells the correct time at least twice a day, right? Be patient with them as well as yourself.

Another thing I considered at one time was joining a support group. Just being around other people with breast cancer and hearing their stories may help you in a way you didn't think it could. Even better, ask a few of your close friends or family to start one for you. A group of your closest friends and family to vent to helps a lot. Whatever you do, just stay calm. You're going through a very traumatic experience, but just keep going. No matter how hard it gets keep pushing. Some final things to keep in mind:

- ✓ Love self first
- ✓ Think & live positive
- ✓ Keep your faith
- ✓ Be encouraged
- ✓ Educate yourself
- ✓ Talk about how you're feeling

- ✓ Make time for yourself
- ✓ Never stop fighting!

I pray that my story will help you get through your storm and encourage you while you stand on that battlefield to fight.

To My Thriving Sisters,

To the woman who is still battling cancer, I would like to say keep your faith, stay strong, and remain focused. At the end of this test, there will be a testimony with your name attached. Don't allow the enemy to hold you down; stay aloft. Who said this would be easy? Not I. As we know, life can sometimes be a struggle, but every time you are faced with an obstacle and get knocked down, get back up, dust yourself off, and continue onward. And for those who need that extra encouragement, I say to you P.U.S.H. = Pray Until Something Happens. Because with each fall, you will become stronger, and your strength will be the best torch you will ever hold.

Love,

Sabrina

P.S. Hold on to this scripture Hebrew 11: 1-3 ~ 1 Now faith is the [a]substance of things hoped for, the [b]evidence of things not seen. 2 For by it the elders obtained a good testimony. 3 By faith we understand that the [c]worlds were framed by the word of God, so that the things which are seen were not made of things which are visible.

BREAST CANCER GLOSSARY

*Parts of this glossary were adapted from the national cancer institute's dictionary of cancer terms and the American Cancer Society's cancer glossary.

**glossary terms relating to radiation therapy adapted from the joint center for radiation therapy's glossary of terms.

A

Absolute Risk

A person's chance of developing a certain disease over a certain time period. The absolute risk of a disease is estimated by looking at a large group of people similar in some way (in terms of age, for example) and counting the number of people in this group who develop the disease over the specified time period. For example, if we followed 100,000 women between the ages of 30 and 34 for one year, about 25 would develop breast cancer. This means the one-year absolute risk of breast cancer for a 30- to 34-year-old woman is 25 per 100,000 women (1 per 4,000 women).

Acupuncture

Use of very thin needles inserted at precise points on

the body that may help control pain and other side effects of treatment or breast cancer itself. It is a type of integrative or complementary therapy.

Adjuvant (Systemic) Therapy

Treatment given in addition to surgery and radiation to treat breast cancer that may have spread to other parts of the body. It may include chemotherapy, targeted therapy and/or hormone therapy.

Alopecia

Hair loss.

Alternative Therapy

Any therapy used instead of standard medical treatments such as surgery, chemotherapy and hormone therapy. Alternative therapies are different from integrative and complementary therapies, which are used in addition to standard treatments. Alternative therapies have not been shown to be effective in treating breast cancer, so it is not safe to use them.

Amenorrhea

The absence or stopping of menstrual periods.

Anesthesia

Loss of feeling or sensation that keeps a person from

feeling pain during surgery or other medical procedures. Local or regional anesthesia may be used for a specific part of the body, such as the breast, by injection of a drug into that area. General anesthesia numbs the entire body and puts a person to sleep with drugs that are injected into a vein or inhaled.

Aneuploid (DNA Ploidy)

The presence of an abnormal number of chromosomes in cancer cells.

Angiogenesis

The growth of new blood vessels that cells need to grow.

Antibody

A protein made by white blood cells that is part of the body's immune system. Each antibody binds to a certain antigen (foreign substance, such as bacteria) and helps the body fight the antigen.

Antibody Therapy

A drug containing an antibody that is specially made to target certain cancer cells.

Anti-carcinogen

An agent that counteracts carcinogens (cancer causing

agents).

Antiemetic

A medicine that prevents or relieves nausea and vomiting.

Antigen

A substance that causes the body to make an immune response. This immune response often involves making antibodies.

Apoptosis

A normal cell process in which a genetically programmed series of events leads to the death of a cell. Cancer cells may block apoptosis.

Areola

The darkly shaded circle of skin surrounding the nipple.

Aromatase Inhibitors
Hormone therapy drugs that lower estrogen levels in the body by blocking aromatase, an enzyme that converts other hormones into estrogen. Aromatase inhibitors are used to treat postmenopausal women with hormone-receptor positive breast cancer.

Aspirate
To remove fluid and a small number of cells.

Atypical Hyperplasia
A benign (not cancer) breast condition where breast cells are growing rapidly (proliferating). The proliferating cells look abnormal under a microscope. Although atypical hyperplasia is not breast cancer, it increases the risk of breast cancer.

Autologous
A blood donation or tissue graft from a person's own body rather than from a donor. For example, autologous breast reconstruction techniques use skin and tissue flaps (grafts) from a person's own body.

Axillary Dissection (Axillary Sampling)
Surgical procedure to remove some or all of the lymph nodes from the underarm area so that the nodes can be examined under a microscope to check whether or not cancer cells are present.

Axillary Lymph Nodes
The lymph nodes in the underarm area.

B

Benign
Not cancerous. Does not invade nearby tissue or spread to other parts of the body.

Benign Breast Conditions (Benign Breast Disease)

Noncancerous conditions of the breast that can result in lumps or other abnormalities. Examples include cysts and fibroadenomas.

Benign Phyllodes Tumor

A rare benign (not cancer) breast condition similar to a fibroadenoma. A lump may be felt, but is usually painless.

Bilateral Prophylactic Mastectomy

Surgery where both breasts are removed to prevent breast cancer from developing.

Biobank (Tissue Repository)

A large collection of tissue samples and medical data that is used for research studies.

Bioimpedance (Bioelectrical Impedance Analysis)

A method of measuring the amount of fluid in body tissues.

Biological Therapy

A therapy that targets something specific to the biology of the cancer cell, as opposed to chemotherapy, which attacks all rapidly dividing cells. Often used to describe therapies that use the immune system to fight cancer (immunotherapy). Trastuzumab (Herceptin) is an example of a biological or targeted therapy agent.

Biomarker
A substance found in blood, other body fluids or tissues that can be measured and is a sign of disease or another process in the body (normal or abnormal). It also may be used to see how well the body responds to a treatment for a disease.

Biopsy
Removal of tissue to be tested for cancer cells.

Bisphosphonates
Drugs used to strengthen bones and decrease the rate of bone fractures and pain due to breast cancer metastases to the bone.

Bone Scan
A test done to check for signs of cancer in the bones. A small amount of radioactive material is injected into the bloodstream. It collects in the bones, especially abnormal areas, and is detected by a scanner. Bone scans can show cancer as well as benign bone diseases (like arthritis).

Boost
Additional dose of radiation to the part of the breast that had the tumor.

BRCA1/BRCA2 Genes (BReast CAncer genes)
Genes that help limit cell growth. A mutation (change) in one of these genes increases a person's

risk of breast, ovarian and certain other cancers.

Brachytherapy
A procedure that uses targeted radiation therapy from inside the tumor bed.

Breast Cancer
An uncontrolled growth of abnormal breast cells.

Breast Cancer Advocacy
Influencing targeted audiences to promote the support of breast cancer issues.

Breast Density
A measure used to describe the relative amounts of fat and tissue in the breasts as seen on a mammogram.

Breast Imaging Reporting and Data System (BI-RADS®)
A system developed by the American College of Radiology to provide a standard way to describe the findings on a mammogram.

Breast Reconstruction
Surgery to restore the look and feel of the breast after mastectomy.

Breast Self-Examination (BSE)
A method that may help women become familiar with the normal look and feel of their breasts. BSE is not recommended as a breast cancer screening tool

because it has not been shown to decrease breast cancer death.

Breast Tomosynthesis (3D Digital Mammography, Digital Tomosynthesis)

A tool that uses a digital mammography machine to take multiple two dimensional (2D) X-ray images of the breast. Computer software combines the multiple 2D images into a three dimensional image. Breast tomosynthesis is not a standard breast cancer screening tool at this time.

C

Calcifications

Deposits of calcium in the breast that appear as bright, white spots on a mammogram. Most calcifications are not cancer. However, tight clusters or lines of tiny calcifications (called microcalcifications) can be a sign of breast cancer.

Cancer

General name for over 100 diseases with uncontrolled cell growth.

Carcinoma in Situ(in Situ Carcinoma)

Condition where abnormal cells are found in the milk ducts or lobules of the breast, but not in the surrounding breast tissue. In situ means "in place." See ductal carcinoma in situ and lobular carcinoma in situ.

Chemoprevention
A drug or combination of drugs used to lower the risk of breast cancer in cancer-free women at higher risk.

Chemotherapy
A drug or combination of drugs that kills cancer cells in various ways.

Clinical Breast Examination (CBE)
A physical exam done by a health care provider to check the look and feel of the breasts and underarm for any changes or abnormalities (such as lumps).

Clinical Trials
Research studies that test the benefits of possible new ways to detect, diagnose, treat or prevent disease. People volunteer to take part in these studies.

Complementary Therapies (Integrative Therapies)
Therapies (such as acupuncture or massage) used in addition to standard medical treatments. Complementary therapies are not used to treat cancer, but they may help improve quality of life and relieve some side effects of treatment or the cancer itself. When complementary therapies are combined with standard medical care, they are often called integrative therapies.

Computer-assisted detection (CAD)
Software developed to help radiologists find suspicious areas on a digital mammogram.

Core Needle Biopsy
A needle biopsy that uses a hollow needle to remove samples of tissue from an abnormal area in the breast.

Co-Survivor
A person who lends support to someone diagnosed with breast cancer, from the time of diagnosis through treatment and beyond. Co-survivors may include family members, spouses or partners, friends, health care providers and colleagues.

CT Scan (Computerized Tomography Scan, Computerized Axial Tomography (CAT) Scan)
A series of pictures created by a computer linked to an X-ray machine. The scan gives detailed internal images of the body.

Cumulative Risk
The sum of a person's chances of developing a disease (like breast cancer) over the course of a lifetime (usually defined as birth up to age 85). For example, the cumulative (lifetime) risk of breast cancer for women is about 1 in 8 (or about 12 percent). This means for every 8 women, one will be diagnosed with breast cancer during her lifetime (up to age 85).

Cyst
A fluid-filled sac.

Cytopathologist
A pathologist who specializes in looking at individual cells. A cytopathologist is needed to interpret the results of fine needle aspiration.

Cytotoxic
Toxic, or deadly, to cells (cell killing). Often used to describe chemotherapy.

D

Definitive Surgery
All of the known tumor is removed and no follow-up surgery is needed.

Diabetic Mastopathy
A rare benign (not cancer) breast condition that consists of small hard masses in the breast. It occurs most often in women with insulin-dependent (type 1) diabetes.

Diagnostic Mammogram
A mammogram used to check symptoms of breast cancer (such as a lump) or an abnormal finding noted on a screening mammogram or clinical breast exam. It involves two or more X-ray views of the breast.

Diagnostic Radiologist (Radiologist)
A health care provider who specializes in the diagnosis of diseases using X-rays.

Diploid (DNA Ploidy)
The presence of a normal number of chromosomes in cancer cells.

Disease-Free Survival Rate
Percent of people alive and without disease at a certain time (often five years or 10 years) after treatment. Those who die from causes other than the disease under study are not included in this measure.

Dose-Dense Therapy
Chemotherapy given over a shorter (more condensed) time period compared to standard therapy. The frequency of treatment sessions is increased, so the length of the treatment period is shortened.

Down-Staging
Lowering the stage of a cancer from its original stage (or the stage it was thought to be). Down-staging occurs most often after a good response to neoadjuvant therapy. Neoadjuvant therapy is chemotherapy or hormone therapy used as a first treatment (before surgery) for some large or advanced breast cancers. Neoadjuvant therapy can shrink a tumor such that it lowers the stage of the breast cancer and a lumpectomy, instead of a mastectomy,

can be done.

Ductal Carcinoma in Situ (DCIS, Intraductal Carcinoma)

A non-invasive breast cancer that begins in the milk ducts of the breast, but has not invaded nearby breast tissue. Also called stage 0 or pre-invasive breast carcinoma.

E

Early Breast Cancer

Cancer that is contained in the breast or has only spread to lymph nodes in the underarm area. This term often describes stage I and stage II breast cancer.

Edema

Excess fluid in body tissues that causes swelling.

Endometrial Cancer

Cancer of the endometrium (the lining of the uterus).

Enzyme

A protein that speeds up biologic reactions in the body.

Epidemiology

The study of the causes and prevention of disease.

Estrogen

A female hormone produced by the ovaries and adrenal glands that is important to reproduction.

Some cancers need estrogen to grow.

Estrogen Receptors
Specific proteins in cells that estrogen hormones attach to. A high number of estrogen receptors on a breast cancer cell often means the cancer cell needs estrogen to grow.

Excisional Biopsy
Surgical procedure that removes the entire abnormal area (plus some surrounding normal tissue) from the breast.

F

False Negative
A test result that incorrectly reports a person is disease-free when she/he actually has the disease.

False Positive
A test result that incorrectly reports a person has a disease when she/he does not have the disease.

Fat Necrosis
A benign (not cancer) breast change in which the breast responds to trauma with a firm, irregular mass, often years after the event. The mass is the result of fatty tissue dying, after either surgery or blunt trauma to the breast. This breast change does not increase risk of breast cancer.

Fibroadenoma

A benign (not cancer) fibrous tumor that may occur at any age, but is more common in young adulthood.

Fibrocystic Condition (Fibrocystic Changes)

A general term used to describe a benign (not cancer) breast condition that may cause painful cysts or lumpy breasts.

First-Line Therapy

The initial (first) therapy used in a person's cancer treatment.

Flow Cytometry

A laboratory test done on tumor tissue to measure the growth rate of the cancer cells and to check if the cells have too much DNA.

Fluorescence In Situ Hybridization (FISH)

A laboratory test done on breast tumor tissue to find out the number of copies of the HER2/neu gene contained in the cancer cells.

Frozen Section

Process where a portion of tissue from a surgical biopsy is frozen so a thin slice can be studied to check for cancer. Frozen section results are only preliminary and always need to be confirmed by other methods.

G

Gail Model (Breast Cancer Risk Assessment Tool)
A tool that uses personal and family history to
estimate a woman's risk of invasive breast cancer.

Galactocele
A milk-filled cyst.

Genes
The part of a cell that contains DNA. The DNA
information in a person's genes is inherited from both
sides of a person's family.

Gene Variant of Uncertain Significance
A gene mutation not currently known to increase
breast cancer risk.

Glandular Tissue (in the breast)
The tissue in the breast that includes the milk
ducts and lobules.

H

**HER2/neu (Human Epidermal Growth Factor
Receptor 2, erbB2)**
A protein involved in cell growth and survival that
appears on the surface of some breast cancer
cells. HER2/neu-negative breast cancers have little or
no HER2/neu protein. HER2/neu-positive breast
cancers have a lot of HER2/neu protein. HER2/neu-

positive tumors can be treated with the targeted therapy drug trastuzumab (Herceptin).

Hospice
A philosophy of care focusing on improving quality of life and easing pain and other symptoms at the end stage of a terminal illness. Hospice care also provides support services to patients and their families.

Hyperplasia (Usual and Atypical Hyperplasia)
A benign (not cancer) breast condition where breast cells are growing rapidly (proliferating). Although hyperplasia is not breast cancer, it increases the risk of breast cancer. In usual hyperplasia, the proliferating cells look normal under a microscope. In atypical hyperplasia, the proliferating cells look abnormal.

I

Immediate Family Member (First-Degree Relative)
A person's mother, father, sister, brother or child.

Immunotherapy
Therapies that use the immune system to fight cancer. These therapies target something specific to the biology of the cancer cell, as opposed to chemotherapy, which attacks all rapidly dividing cells. See Biological Therapy.

Immunohistochemistry (IHC)
A laboratory test done on tumor tissue to detect the

amount of HER2/neu protein on the surface of the cancer cells.

Implant (Breast Implant)
An "envelope" containing silicone, saline or both, that is used to restore the breast form after a mastectomy (or for other cosmetic reasons).

Incidence
The number of new cases of a disease that develop in a specific time period.

Incisional Biopsy
Surgical biopsy that removes only part of the tumor.

Inflammatory Breast Cancer (IBC)
A rare and aggressive form of invasive breast cancer. Its main symptoms are swelling (inflammation) and redness of the breast. The skin on the breast may look dimpled, like the skin of an orange, and may be warm to the touch.

Informed Consent
The process through which a person learns about the possible benefits and side effects of a treatment plan and then accepts or declines the treatment. The person is usually asked to sign a consent form, but may stop the treatment at any time and get other medical care.

Intraductal
Within the milk duct. Intraductal can describe a benign (not cancerous) or malignant (cancerous) process.

Intraductal Hyperplasia
An excess of cells growing within the milk ducts of the breast.

Intraductal Papilloma (Ductal Papilloma)
Small, benign (not cancer) growths that begin in the ducts of the breast and usually cannot be felt. Symptoms include a bloody or clear nipple discharge.

Invasive Breast Cancer
Cancer that has spread from the original location (milk ducts or lobules) into the surrounding breast tissue and possibly into the lymph nodes and other parts of the body. Invasive ductal cancer begins in the milk ducts. Invasive lobular cancer begins in the lobules of the breast.

K

Ki-67 Rate
A common way to measure proliferation rate. The more cells the Ki-67 antibody attaches to on a tissue sample, the more likely the tumor cells are to grow and divide rapidly.

L

Lesion
Area of abnormal tissue.

Lifetime Risk
The chance of developing a disease (like breast cancer) over the course of a lifetime (usually defined as birth up to age 85). For example, the lifetime risk of breast cancer for women is 1 in 8 (or about 12 percent). This means for every 8 women, one will be diagnosed with breast cancer during her lifetime (up to age 85).

Linear Accelerator
The device used during radiation therapy to direct X-rays into the body.

Liquid biopsy
A test that measures levels of circulating tumor cells or circulating tumor DNA in the blood. These tests are under study for use in monitoring metastatic breast cancer. Although the term includes the word "biopsy," these tests are not used for breast cancer diagnosis.

Local Anesthetic
Anesthesia that only numbs the tissue in a certain area. See Anesthesia.

Local Treatment

Treatment that focuses on getting rid of the cancer from a certain (local) area. In breast cancer, the local area includes the breast, the chest wall and lymph nodes in the underarm area (axillary nodes). Local treatment for breast cancer includes surgery with or without radiation therapy.

Localized Breast Cancer

Cancer that is contained in the breast and has not spread to nearby tissue, lymph nodes or other organs.

Locally Advanced Breast Cancer (Stage III Breast Cancer)

Cancer that has spread beyond the breast to the skin or chest wall, but not to distant organs like the lungs or liver. It also refers to a tumor that is larger than five centimeters (about two inches) in size.

Local Recurrence (Recurrence)

The return of cancer to the same breast or to the same side chest wall.

Lump

Any mass in the breast or elsewhere in the body.

Lumpectomy (Breast Conserving Surgery)

Surgery that removes only part of the breast — the part containing and closely surrounding the tumor.

Lymph Nodes (Lymph Glands)
Small groups of immune cells that act as filters for the lymphatic system. Clusters of lymph nodes are found in the underarms, groin, neck, chest and abdomen.

Lymph Node Status
Shows whether or not cancer has spread to the lymph nodes. Lymph node-positive means that cancer has spread to the lymph nodes. Lymph node-negative means that cancer has not spread to the lymph nodes. See Lymph Nodes.

Lymphatic System
The network of lymph nodes and vessels in the body.

Lymphedema
Swelling due to poor draining of lymph fluid that can occur after surgery to remove lymph nodes or after radiation therapy to the area. Most often occurs in the upper limbs (arm, hands or fingers), but can occur in other parts of the body.

M

Malignant
Cancerous.

Mammary Duct Ectasia
A benign (not cancer) breast condition resulting from inflammation (swelling) and enlargement of the ducts behind the nipple. Often there are no symptoms,

but calcifications seen on a mammogram may point to its presence. No treatment is needed if the woman is not having symptoms (burning, pain or itching in the nipple area).

Mammary Glands
The breast glands that produce milk.

Mammogram
An X-ray image of the breast.

Mastectomy
Surgical removal of the breast. The exact procedure depends on the diagnosis. See Total Mastectomy and Modified Radical Mastectomy.

Mastitis
An inflammation (swelling) of the breast usually occurring during breastfeeding. Symptoms include pain, nipple discharge, fever, redness and hardness over an area of the breast.

Medical Oncologist
A physician specializing in the treatment of cancer using chemotherapy, hormone therapy and targeted therapy.

Melatonin
Hormone made by the pineal gland in the brain. It is an important part of the body's internal timing system.

Metastasis

The spread of cancer to other organs through the lymphatic and/or circulatory system. Metastases is the plural of metastasis.

Metastasize

When cancer cells spread to other organs through the lymphatic and/or circulatory system.

Metastatic breast cancer

Breast cancer that has spread beyond the breast to other organs in the body (most often the bones, lungs, liver or brain). Metastatic breast cancer is not a specific type of breast cancer, but rather the most advanced stage (stage IV) of breast cancer.

Microcalcifications

Small, clustered deposits of calcium in the breast that may be seen on a mammogram. These may or may not be related to breast cancer.

Modified Radical Mastectomy

Surgical removal of the breast, the lining of the chest muscles and some of the lymph nodes in the underarm area. Used to treat early and locally advanced breast cancer.

Monoclonal Antibodies

Immune proteins that can locate and bind to cancer cells. They can be used alone or they can be used to deliver drugs, toxins or radioactive material directly to tumor cells. Trastuzumab (Herceptin) is an example of a monoclonal antibody used to treat breast cancer.

Multifocal Tumors (Multicentric Tumors)
One or more tumors that develop from the original breast tumor.

Multimodality Therapy
Use of two or more treatment methods (such as surgery, radiation therapy, chemotherapy, hormone therapy and targeted therapy) in combination or one after the other to get the best results.

N

Neoadjuvant Chemotherapy (Induction Chemotherapy, Primary Chemotherapy, Preoperative Chemotherapy)
Chemotherapy used as a first treatment. Often used for large or locally-advanced cancers to shrink tumors before surgery.

Neoadjuvant Hormone Therapy
Hormone therapy used as a first treatment. Often used for large or locally-advanced cancers to shrink tumors before surgery.

Neoadjuvant Therapy (Preoperative Therapy)
Chemotherapy or hormone therapy used as a first treatment. Often used for large or locally-advanced

cancers to shrink tumors before surgery.

Neoplasia
Abnormal growth.

Neoplasm
Excess number of cells in a mass that can be either benign (not cancerous) or malignant (cancerous).

Nipple-Sparing Mastectomy
A breast reconstruction procedure that removes the tumor and margins as well as the fat and other tissue in the breast, but leaves the nipple and areola intact.

Node-Negative (Lymph Node-Negative)
Cancer that has not spread to the lymph nodes. See Lymph Node Status.

Node-Positive (Lymph Node-Positive)
Cancer that has spread to the lymph nodes. See Lymph Node Status.

Non-Invasive
1. In treatment, describes a procedure that does not penetrate the skin (or any body opening) with a needle or other instrument.

2. In breast cancer pathology, describes a cancer that has not spread beyond the ducts or lobules where it began (see Carcinoma in Situ).

Nonpalpable

Describes a breast lump or abnormal area that cannot be felt but can be seen on an imaging test (such as a mammogram).

Normal Tissue

Cells that are cancer-free.

Nuclear Medicine Imaging of the Breast (Molecular Breast Imaging)

A technique under study for use in the early detection of breast cancer. Nuclear medicine imaging uses short-term radioactive agents given through an IV. Cancer cells absorb these agents and can be imaged with a special camera. Nuclear medicine imaging is not a standard breast cancer screening tool. Breast-specific gamma imaging and scintimammography are types of nuclear medicine imaging.

O

Oncologist

The physician in charge of planning and overseeing cancer treatment.

Oophorectomy

Surgical removal of the ovaries.

Osteoporosis

A condition marked by a loss of bone mass and density that causes bones to become fragile.

Over-Diagnosis

Diagnosis that occurs when a mammogram finds ductal carcinoma in situ (DCIS) or a small, invasive breast cancer that would have never caused symptoms or problems if left untreated. These breast cancers may never grow or a person may die from another cause before the breast cancer becomes a problem.

Over-Treatment

Treatment for ductal carcinoma in situ (DCIS) or a small, invasive breast cancer that would have never caused symptoms or problems if left untreated.

Overall Survival (Overall Survival Rate, Survival)

The percentage of people alive for a certain period of time after diagnosis with a disease (such as breast cancer) or treatment for a disease.

P

Paget Disease of the Breast (Paget Disease of the Nipple)

A rare cancer in the skin of the nipple or in the skin closely surrounding the nipple that is usually, but not always, found with an underlying breast cancer (ductal in situ carcinoma or invasive breast cancer). In these cases, the tumor grows from underneath the nipple and breaks out onto the surface of the nipple.

Palliative Therapy (Palliative Care, Palliation)
Care focused on relieving or preventing symptoms (like pain) rather than treating disease.

Palpable
Describes a breast lump or abnormal area that can be felt during a clinical breast exam.

Pathologic Response
A measure describing how much of the tumor is left in the breast and lymph nodes after neoadjuvant (before surgery) therapy. The pathologic response gives some information about prognosis. A complete pathologic response means there is no invasive cancer in the tissue removed during breast surgery.

Pathologist
The physician who uses a microscope to study the breast tissue and lymph nodes removed during biopsy or surgery and determines whether or not the cells contain cancer.

Peri-Menopause
The time in a woman's life prior to menopause when menstrual periods become irregular and some menopausal symptoms may begin.

Peripherally Inserted Central Catheter (PICC)
A small tube used to deliver medicine to the body through a vein. Instead of being reinserted for each use, a PICC is left in place to allow access for a long period of time (weeks to months).

Personalized Medicine
Using information about a person's genes, the tumor's genes, molecular characteristics of the tumor and the environment to prevent, diagnose and treat disease (such as the use of targeted therapies).This may also be known as precision medicine.

PET (Positron Emission Tomography)
A procedure where a short-term radioactive sugar is given through an IV so that a scanner can show which parts of the body are consuming more sugar. Cancer cells tend to consume more sugar than normal cells do. PET is sometimes used as part of breast cancer diagnosis or treatment, but is not used for breast cancer screening.

Pharmacogenomics (Pharmacogenetics)
The study of the way genes affect a person's response to drugs to help predict which drugs may offer him/her the most benefit.

Phyllodes Tumor
A rare sarcoma (cancer of the soft tissue) in the breast.

Pituitary Gland
A part of the brain that controls growth and other glands in the body, such as the ovaries.

Placebo
An inactive medicine sometime used to have a comparison to a new drug in a clinical study. May be called a "sugar pill."

Pooled Analysis
A method for collecting the individual data from a group of studies, combining them into one large set of data and then analyzing the data as if they came from one big study.

Precision Medicine
Using information about a person's genes, the tumor's genes, molecular characteristics of the tumor and the environment to prevent, diagnose and treat disease (such as the use of targeted therapies). This may also be known as personalized medicine.

Primary Tumor
The original cancer.

Progesterone
A hormone made by the body that is important in menstrual cycles and pregnancy. May be made in a laboratory (called progestin) and used in birth control

pills, menopausal hormone therapy and other types of hormone treatment.

Progesterone Receptor
Specific proteins on cells that progesterone hormones attach to. A high number of progesterone receptors on a breast cancer cell often means the cancer cell needs progesterone to grow.

Progestin
Any substance (laboratory-made or natural) that has some or all of the effects of progesterone in the body.

Prognosis
The expected or probable outcome or course of a disease (the chance of recovery).

Prognostic Factors
Factors (such as tumor type, size and grade) that help determine prognosis.

Progression
The growth or spread of cancer, with or without treatment.

Progression-Free Survival
The length of time a person lives with cancer (such as metastatic breast cancer) before the cancer grows or spreads.

Prophylactic Mastectomy
Preventive surgery where one or both breasts are

removed in order to prevent breast cancer. When both breasts are removed the procedure is called bilateral prophylactic mastectomy.

Prosthetic (Breast Prosthetic, Prosthesis)
An artificial breast form that can be worn under clothing after a mastectomy.

Q

Quadrantectomy
Surgery where one quadrant or 25 percent of the breast is removed.

Quality of Care
Measures of how well breast cancer is treated and how well a person is cared for during and after treatment.

Quality of Life
A measure of a person's well-being and his/her overall enjoyment of life.

Quartiles
Categories of an exposure (like body weight or exercise) based on four equal parts of the total number of people in the study.

R

RAD (dose of radiation)

Short for "radiation absorbed dose." This term describes the amount of radiation absorbed by the tissues. One RAD is equal to one centigray. See Centigray.

Radial Scars (Complex Sclerosing Lesions)
A benign (not cancer) breast condition with a core of connective tissue fibers. Ducts and lobules grow out from this core.

Radiation Oncologist
A physician specializing in the treatment of cancer using targeted, high energy X-rays.

Radiation Therapy (Radiotherapy)
Treatment given by a radiation oncologist that uses targeted, high energy X-rays to kill cancer cells.

Radical Mastectomy (Halsted Radical)
Surgical removal of the breast, chest muscles and underarm lymph nodes. Used only when the breast tumor has spread to the chest muscles.

Radiologist
A physician who reads and interprets X-rays, mammograms and other scans related to diagnosis or follow-up. Radiologists also perform needle biopsy and wire localization procedures.

Raloxifene
A drug first used to treat osteoporosis and now also

used to lower the risk of breast cancer in postmenopausal women at high risk.

Recurrence (Relapse)
Return of cancer. Local recurrence is the return of cancer to the same breast or the same side chest wall. Distant recurrence is the return of cancer that has spread to other parts of the body, such as the lungs, liver, bones or brain. See Metastases.

Regimen
A treatment plan.

Regional Lymph Nodes
In breast cancer, the axillary (in the underarm area) lymph nodes, infraclavicular (under the collarbone) lymph nodes, supraclavicular (above the collarbone) lymph nodes and internal mammary nodes.
See Lymph Nodes.

Regression
The shrinking of a tumor.

Retrospective Study
A study where both the exposure (such as alcohol use) and the outcome (such as breast cancer) occur before the start of the study.

Risk (of disease)
Probability (chance) of disease developing in a person during a specified time period.

S

Saline
A saltwater solution similar to that found in IV fluids. Saline can be used to fill a breast implant.

Scalp Cooling
The use of a cap filled with a chilled substance during chemotherapy. Scalp cooling is under study as a technique for reducing hair loss due to chemotherapy.

Schedules
The different combinations and timing for chemotherapy and other drugs.

Sclerosing Adenosis
Small, benign (not cancer) breast lumps caused by enlarged lobules. The lumps may be felt and may be painful.

Screening
A test or procedure used to find cancer or a benign (not cancer) condition in a person who does not have any known problems or symptoms.

Screening Mammogram
A test used to find early signs of breast cancer in a woman who does not have any known breast problems or symptoms.

Second Primary Tumor
A second breast cancer that develops in a different

location from the first. This is different from a local recurrence, which is the return of the first breast cancer.

Sentinel Node Biopsy
The surgical removal and testing of the sentinel node(s) (first axillary node(s) in the underarm area filtering lymph fluid from the tumor site) to see if the node(s) contains cancer cells.

Silicone Gel
Medical-grade, solid form of silicone used for breast implants. Silicone implants can mimic the feel of a natural breast better than saline implants.

Skin-Sparing Mastectomy
A procedure that surgically removes the breast, but keeps intact as much of the skin that surrounds the breast as possible. This skin can then be used in breast reconstruction to cover a tissue flap or an implant instead of having to use skin from other parts of the body.

Stage of Cancer (Cancer Stage)
A way to indicate the extent of the cancer within the body. The most widely used staging method for breast cancer is the TNM system, which uses Tumor size, lymph Node status and the absence or presence of Metastases to classify breast cancers.

Staging (Cancer Staging)
Doing tests to learn the extent of the cancer within the body (the cancer's stage 0 to IV). Knowing a cancer's stage helps determine what treatment is needed and how effective this treatment may be in getting rid of the disease and prolonging life.

Standard Treatment (Standard of Care)
The usual treatment of a disease or condition currently in widespread use and considered to be of proven effectiveness on the basis of scientific evidence and past experience.

Stereotactic Mammography
Three-dimensional mammography used to guide a needle biopsy.

Surgeon
Physician who performs any surgery, including surgical biopsies and other procedures related to breast cancer.

Surgical Oncologist
A physician specializing in the treatment of cancer using surgical procedures.

Survivors (Breast Cancer Survivors)
People with a history of breast cancer, from the time of diagnosis to the end of their lives.

Survivorship
The emotional and physical health, life and care of a breast cancer survivor from the time of diagnosis until the end of life.

Systemic (Adjuvant) Treatment
treatment given in addition to surgery and radiation to treat breast cancer that may have spread to other parts of the body. It may include chemotherapy, targeted therapy and/or hormone therapy.

T

Tamoxifen (Nolvadex)
A hormone therapy drug (taken in pill form) used to treat early and advanced stage breast cancers that are hormone receptor-positive. These breast cancers need estrogen to grow. Tamoxifen stops or slows the growth of these tumors by blocking estrogen from attaching to hormone receptor in the cancer cells.

Targeted Therapy
Drug therapies designed to attack specific molecular agents or pathways involved in the development of cancer. Trastuzumab (Herceptin) is an example of a targeted therapy used to treat breast cancer.

Total Mastectomy (Simple Mastectomy)
Surgical removal of the breast but no other tissue or nodes. Used for the treatment of ductal carcinoma in

...tu and, in some cases, breast cancer recurrence. Also used in prophylactic mastectomy.

Trastuzumab (Herceptin)

A drug that is a specially made antibody that targets cancer cells with a lot of the protein called HER2/neu on their surfaces. When attached to the HER2/neu protein, trastuzumab slows or stops the growth of the cancer cells. Trastuzumab is used to treat HER2/neu-positive breast cancer. Herceptin is the brand name for trastuzumab.

Triple Negative Breast Cancer

A breast cancer that is estrogen receptor-negative, progesterone receptor-negative and HER2/neu-negative. These factors limit treatment choices. Most triple negative tumors are basal-like tumors. These breast cancers tend to be aggressive and are more common in African American women.

Tumor

An abnormal growth or mass of tissue that may be benign (not cancerous) or malignant (cancerous).

Tumor Grade

Describes how closely cancer cells look like normal cells. Grade 1 tumors have cells that are slow-growing and look the most like normal cells. Grade 3 tumors have cells that are fast-growing and look very abnormal. Grade 2 tumors fall in between grade 1 and grade 3.

Tumor Marker

A substance found in blood that may be a sign of metastatic breast cancer. Tumor markers are found in both normal cells and cancer cells, but they are made in larger amounts by cancer cells. A tumor marker may help indicate metastatic breast cancer treatment activity. The term tumor marker may also be used more broadly to refer to characteristics of tumor cells such as hormone receptors.

Tumor Profiling (Gene Expression Profiling)

Tests that give information about thousands of genes in cancer cells. Specific genes (or combinations of genes) may give information useful in prognosis and in making treatment decisions.

Two-Step Procedure

Biopsy and further surgical treatment done at two separate times.

Tyrosine-Kinase Inhibitors

A class of drugs that target enzymes important for cell functions (called tyrosine-kinase enzymes). These drugs can block tyrosine-kinase enzymes at many points along the cancer growth pathway.

U

Ultrasound (Sonogram)
Diagnostic test that uses sound waves to make images of tissues and organs. Tissues of different densities reflect sound waves differently.

Usual Hyperplasia
A benign (not cancer) breast condition where breast cells are growing rapidly (proliferating). The proliferating cells look normal under a microscope. Although usual hyperplasia is not breast cancer, it increases the risk of breast cancer.

V

Vaginal Atrophy (Atrophic Vaginitis)
Vaginal dryness.

W

Wire Localization (Needle Localization)
Insertion of a very thin wire into the breast to highlight the location of an abnormal area so that it can be removed during biopsy or lumpectomy.

X

X-ray
Radiation that, at low levels, can be used to make images of the inside of the body. For example, a

mammogram is an X-ray image of the breast. At high levels of radiation, X-rays can be used in cancer treatment.

SUPPORT & RESOURCE ORGANIZATIONS

4th Angel - Patient and Caregiver Mentoring Program
Offers telephone support programs for women living
with breast cancer and their caregivers.
www.4thangel.org/

After Breast Cancer Diagnosis (ABCD)
Offers online and telephone support for people
diagnosed with breast cancer and their loved ones.
1-800-977-4121
www.abcdbreastcancersupport.org

American Cancer Society
Find local support programs and services.
www.cancer.org/treatment/support-programs-and-services.html

American Cancer Society - Cancer Survivors Network
Offers an online community where people diagnosed
with breast cancer and caregivers share their
experiences and recommend helpful resources.
www.csn.cancer.org/

American Cancer Society - Reach to Recovery
Connects people newly diagnosed with breast cancer
and their families with trained volunteers (who are

breast cancer survivors) in their area.
1-800-227-2345
www.cancer.org/treatment/support-programs-and-services/reach-to-recovery.html

Association of Cancer Online Resources
Find an online support group.
www.acor.org/

Cancer and Careers
Find information for working women with cancer.
www.cancerandcareers.org/

Cancer Support Community
(formerly Gilda's Club Worldwide and The Wellness Community) Offers in-person, online and telephone support for people diagnosed with breast cancer and their loved ones.
1-888-793-9355
www.cancersupportcommunity.org

CancerCare
Find an online support group.
www.cancercare.org/

CancerConnect
Find an online support group.
www.cancerconnect.com

CaringBridge
Offers personal, protected sites with multiple privacy settings where people can stay connected during any type of health event. An online planner can help family and friends coordinate care and helpful tasks.
www.caringbridge.org

Here for the Girls
Offers online and in-person support for young women affected by breast cancer.
www.hereforthegirls.org/support/

Imerman Angels
Offers online support programs for women and men living with cancer and their caregivers.
www.imermanangels.org/

Living Beyond Breast Cancer
Find information on breast cancer support and care.
www.lbbc.org/

Mautner Project of Whitman-Walker Health
Offers online and telephone support programs for lesbian, bisexual and transgender individuals living with cancer, and their partners.
1-866-MAUTNER (1-866-628-8637)
www.whitman-walker.org/service/community-health/mautner-project/

SHARE Cancer Support
Offers telephone support groups for women newly diagnosed with breast cancer and women who have lymphedema.
1-844-ASK-SHARE (1-844-275-7427)
www.sharecancersupport.org/

Susan G. Kormen
For breast health or breast cancer information, please call the Breast Care Helpline
1-877 GO KOMEN (1-877- 465- 6636)
helpline@komen.org
https://ww5.komen.org/

Unite for Her
Unite for HER is committed to helping women diagnosed with breast cancer navigate their way through treatment by providing complementary therapies designed to promote physical and emotional wellness.
https://uniteforher.org/

Young Survival Coalition
Provides support programs (online and telephone) for young women diagnosed with breast cancer, and a resource kit for young women newly diagnosed with breast cancer.
www.youngsurvival.org/

ABOUT SABRINA L. MOORE

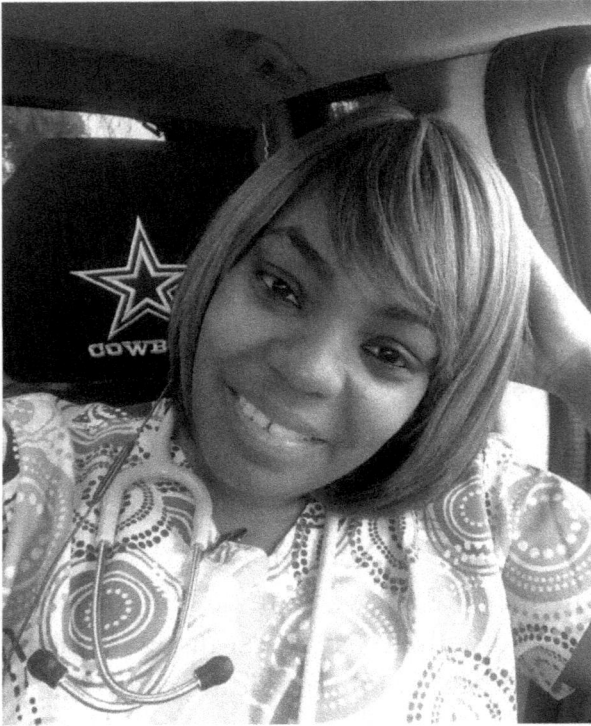

Born and raised in North Philadelphia, Pennsylvania, Sabrina Moore is a 39-year-old Breast Cancer Survivor and mother to three beautiful children, two of which are biologically hers. She is also helping to raise her goddaughter. Sabrina is the youngest of ten children and very family-oriented. Her mother, who Sabrina likes to refer to as her backbone, has especially played an important role in Sabrina's life, giving her the encouragement she needed to stay determined and never give up.

Sabrina worked in the medical community for ten years at Quality Community Health Care. After becoming her maternal grandmother's caregiver and then becoming sick herself with cancer, Sabrina resigned from her position as a Dental Billing Specialist. Having a passion to help others, her dream has always been to become a nurse, and she is currently going to school to fulfill that dream and become a registered nurse who provides care to those in Hospice care.

Sabrina attended Strawberry Mansion High School but graduated from Northeast Learning Center in Philadelphia. Afterward, she earned her Medical Assistant Certification from All-State Career School and is currently working for Patriot Home Care as a caregiver.

Sabrina's hobbies include cooking, shopping, having fun, and caring for others. She is also an active member of Living Beyond Breast Cancer.

Do You Know Others In Their Own Way??

Share This Book!
Order More Copies

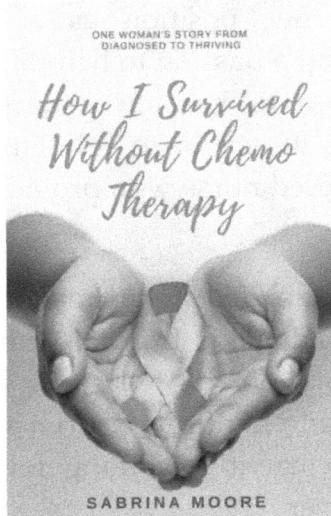

ONE WOMAN'S STORY FROM
DIAGNOSED TO THRIVING

How I Survived
Without Chemo
Therapy

SABRINA MOORE

Retail Price $12.99
Special Quantity Discounts

5-99 Books	$10.95 each
100-999 Books	$9.95 each
1000+ Books	$6.95 each

To Place An Order Contact:
sweettee927@gmail.com